The Skinny

The Skinny

What Every
Skinny Woman Knows
About Dieting
(And Won't Tell You!)

PATRICIA MARX AND
SUSAN SISTROM

A Dell Trade Paperback

Library of Congress Cataloging in Publication Data
Marx, Patricia (Patricia A.)
The skinny : what every skinny woman knows (and won't tell
you!) / Patricia Marx and Susan Sistrom.
p.   cm.
ISBN: 0-440-50855-X
1. Weight loss.   2. Women—Health and hygiene.
I. Sistrom, Susan.   II. Title.
RM222.2.M3695   1999   98-54824
613'.04244—dc21   CIP

To Aunt Jemima, Sara Lee,
Colonel Sanders, Ben & Jerry,
and Baby Ruth.

And, of course, Twiggy.

And, of course, our moms.

ACKNOWLEDGMENTS

We'd like to thank Jim Traub and Buffy Easton, at whose dinner party the idea of doing a book together first dawned on us (during dessert).

Our thanks to Richard Pine and all the great people at Dell, especially Diane Bartoli, Kristin Cauthorn, Robyn Forkos, and our wonderful editor and publisher, Leslie Schnur.

Most of what we know we learned from our friends and our Skinny Lunch companions. Thanks to:

Diane Asadorian • Susan Becker • Sarah Baldwin-Beneich • Lisa Birnbach • Helen Bransford • Jeff Brown • Sue Borowitz • Karen Brooks • Sasha Buhler • E. Jean Caroll • Joyce Caruso • Mary Beth Caschetta • Susan Casey • Phoebe Cates • Roz Chast • Bill Cohan • Patti Cohen • Jeff Conti • Sarah Crichton • Suzi Dietz • Jean Doumanian • Julie Flanders • Deb Futter • Laura Galen • Marjorie Galen • Ruthie Galen • Lynn Geller • Judith Gittenstein • Amy Godine • Louise Godine • Karen Goldsmith • Elaine Goldsmith Thomas • Gail Gregg • J. Halpern • Jane Hamblin • Amy Handelsman • Elizabeth Hayt • Lynn Hirschberg • Ann Hodgman • Phoebe Hoban • Joan Hornig • Muffin Humes • Julie Huss • Dee Ito • Rebecca Johnson • John Johnson • Marilyn Johnson • Suzy Johnson • J. S. Kaplan • Lisa Klausner • Victoria Klein • Cynthia Kling • Karen Klopp • Carol Kramer • Alex Kuczynski • Corby Kummer • Tajlei Levis • Gordon Lish • Leslie Goodman-Malamuth • Karen Marta • Jane Martin • Joy Marx • Sarah Jane Marx •

Richard Marx · Pearson Marx · Martha McCully ·
Celia McGee · Doug McGrath · Nell Minow ·
Mary Murray · Bill Ndini · Sara Nelson ·
Sheila Nevins · Lucille Nieporent · Sue Nirenberg ·
David Orlean · Debra Orlean · Annette Osher ·
Sarah Paley · Lynne Pepall · Andy Port ·
Francine Prose · Rebecca Prussen · David Rakoff ·
Linda Ratner · Kathy Rich · Victoria Roberts ·
Jennifer Rogers · Marissa Rothkoph · Alison Rose ·
Nina Rosenstein · Victoria Rostow · Sally Sampson ·
Wendy Sarasohn · Irene Sax · Wendy Shanker ·
Susan Shapiro · Judith Shulevitz · Leslie Simitch ·
Dorothy Sistrom · Peter Sistrom · Lynn Snowden ·
Jeff Sonnenfeld · Jane Sosland · Anne Spieleberg ·
Susan Squire · Cyndi Stivers · Sarah Stuart ·
Sarah Thyer · Mary Turner · Mim Udovitch ·
Janet Unglass · Patricia Volk · Linda Winer ·
Lizz Winstead · Maxine Wishner

Special thanks to our medical team—Manny
Alvarez, David McDowell, Lorraine Eyerman, Susan
Fried, Janet Kamin, Jeff Kaplan, Ann Kelly, and Carey
Willis.

And finally, we are grateful to our tireless and slender researcher, Dan Kaufman, who left no calorie un-
turned.

Contents

The Skinny

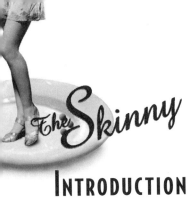

INTRODUCTION

One night over dinner, we were discussing the expansion of NATO, Kantian epistemology, and the likelihood that the universe is composed of tiny superstrings that stretch across ten dimensions. No, actually, we were not. We were busy contemplating the bread basket, trying to decide which had more calories—the corn bread or the sourdough. In other words, we were talking about a subject we know by heart: dieting.

That night, we stopped mid-calorie-count to consider the subject. We computed that over the last twenty years, we had lost a combined total of roughly 23,000 pounds, gained roughly 23,001. We had spent 40–60 percent of our waking hours and 60–80 percent of our sleeping hours consumed by thoughts about our weight. We had been Low-Fat/High-Carbohydrate; High-Fat/Low-Protein; High-Everything; Low-Everything. One us had even been on the All-Artificial-Baco-Bit Diet (by the way, it didn't work). We realized that we could recite calorie counts the way many men could recite batting averages (and they say women don't like math!). We couldn't recall the plots of most movies we'd seen, but we could definitely recall whether we'd eaten popcorn while we watched and whether it was buttered or not. We knew which pair of pants to wear if we were five pounds up or five pounds down. We could stay up all night comparing artificial sweeteners.

We were diet geniuses.

And so are most women. It was a pity, we thought, that all this knowledge wasn't in the public domain. We resolved not to write a "diet" book touting our *Revolutionary Plan* ("Only eat foods beginning with letters in the first half of the alphabet and only on days of the month that are divisible by three!"). Instead, we wanted to compile the folklore and wisdom of women who care about their weight. We decided to talk to as many people as possible, starting with experts. Then, we would move on to those who really know something about losing weight: people Who've Done It. We held a series of lunches—we dubbed them The Skinny Lunches—with our friends and their friends and *their* friends to trade secrets, tips, and strategies we'd all picked up in the field.

We weren't looking for magic (though it would have been nice). After all, weighing less is basically a function of eating less and exercising more (as the diet books say); but *that* is not so easy to achieve (as the diet books forget to mention). Over the years, we had developed our own methods to psyche ourselves into losing weight, or at least not gaining. We perfected the "Make It Look Big" technique of preparing a small amount of food to make it look bulkier. We brush our teeth soon after dinner to prevent late-night snacking. When traveling, we call ahead to the hotel and request a room without a minibar. We hoped to collect many more tricks like these.

We wanted to find out what really works, not what

diet books tell you works. Those books, written by doctors, nutritionists, biochemists, and diet gurus seemed full of scientific theories that contradicted each other. Protein was the key to weight loss one day, glucose the next day, brown fat after that. We were also bored by magazine diets that rehashed the obvious: "Take the stairs instead of the elevator." "Drink eight glasses of water a day." "Try to cut back on fats." We already knew not to consume lard. We were seeking answers to more advanced questions. Tight jeans or loose jeans? Breakfast or not? Should you weigh yourself? How many pounds can you lose by breaking up with a boyfriend?

The Skinny Lunches were the tastiest part of our research. Of course, organizing a meal to talk about not eating presents challenges, especially in our hometown, New York City—the Eating Capital of the Country. It would have been cruel to hold the Skinny Lunches over a marbled sirloin at Peter Luger's Steak House or anywhere within sight of The Little Pie Company. But fortunately, New York's excess of restaurants includes some that have low-caloric dishes on the menu: The Four Seasons with its spa cuisine, Orso with its lean tuna and grilled vegetables, and Coco Pazzo with its cod poached in broth.

Still, there was the problem of diplomacy. Lest anyone interpret our invitation to a Skinny Lunch as a message that we considered her overweight, we overcompensated with abundant praise: "You know, you're very trim. . . . I bet you're the trimmest person I know. . . . I've actually always wondered how you stay so trim. . . . Of course, you're probably one of those people who is naturally trim, right? Oh, gee, it just occurs to me that I'm writing a book about trimness.

By any chance, are you free for lunch Thursday at one o'clock?"

To our surprise and delight, nearly every woman we approached felt she had a lot to say about the topic of weight. "I'd love to come," was the typical response, "but of course, I'll be the fattest one there." In fact, the only people who seemed to be offended were those we had regarded as too nonchalant about their bodies to participate in a Skinny Lunch. "I can't believe you don't think I'm neurotic enough to attend!" one friend complained to us, running through all the odd-ball diets she had tried in her youth.

The lunches were enlightening and a lot of fun, and not only for those involved. Toward the end of one lunch, a woman at the next table stopped by before leaving the restaurant to tell us how much she had enjoyed eavesdropping on our conversation. Waiters typically lingered after serving our food, listening in on, for instance, our theories about why dogs always choose Häagen-Dazs vanilla ice cream over steak (this preference was a "fact," according to one woman, whose father had experimentally proven it in his kitchen). We collected all sorts of advice, ranging from the sensible—"If you are dieting and have kids in the house, buy cookies you don't like."—to the, well, inspired—"Put ice in your water because cold water burns more calories than lukewarm water."

Not everyone at our lunches considered herself a dieter, at least in the cottage-cheese-and-half-a-grapefruit sense of the word. But just about every woman had devised over the years a particular system of eating and exercise to maintain some control over her weight. For some, the rules are rigid ("Never eat before three-thirty in the afternoon."); others are

4

kinder to themselves ("No alcohol, except beer doesn't count as liquor and, on special occasions, neither does wine."); and still other women had rules so relaxed they hardly qualified as rules ("I make sure I never deprive myself of anything.").

So what works? We concluded that losing weight is a very individualized enterprise. The women we heard from at the Skinny Lunches, in buffet lines, on the StairMaster beside us at the gym, and long ago during late-night talks in our dorm rooms had all gathered bits and pieces from many conventional diets and cobbled them together to form something personal. The one-size-fits-all-diets found in diet books do not work for everyone in the world, we were told again and again. What really works is a more mix-and-match approach. The methods and motivations of the women we talked to were various, and often, so were their goals. In the following pages, you will find their insights and recommendations, along with quite a few of our own that we have picked up on the road to losing our 23,000 pounds.

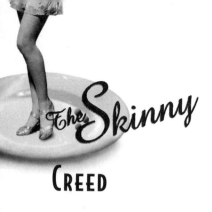

The Skinny

CREED

WE BELIEVE THAT WOMEN WHO DIET KNOW MORE THAN THE DOCTORS WHO STUDY THEM

Come up with any theory about how to lose weight and there is already a diet book to prove it—and still another to disprove it. The more diet literature we read, the more we become convinced that doctors and nutritionists as a group know very little, though they express it with absolute certainty. Year after year, one fad replaces another until there are no fads left and they have to repeat the cycle. Hence, *The Royal Canadian Air Force Diet* goes away and comes back reincarnated as the *Stillman Diet* which then returns years later as the *Diabetes Solution Diet*. In 1972, millions of Americans read *Dr. Atkins' Diet Revolution* and ate hamburgers, eggs, and cream. In 1997, even more Americans read *Dr. Atkins' New Diet Revolution* and returned to hamburgers, eggs, and cream. But a version of those diets had already been promoted in 1863 by a Mr. William Banting, undertaker for the English royal family, whose *Banting's Letter on Corpulence* encouraged a diet with little or no carbohydrates.

On the other hand, there are the women who have been out in the field, doing research, as it were. These are the women who travel to third world countries to drop a quick 8 pounds. (See The Skinny on

Travel.) The women who steer their dates to expensive restaurants because there, the food tends to be less fattening. (See The Skinny on Eating Out.) The women who deal with sudden urges to overeat by painting their fingernails so they can't put food into their mouths. The women who swallow hard-boiled eggs whole to fill themselves up. (See The Skinny on Oddball Tips.) The women who know how to look skinny in a photo even if they are fat. (See The Skinny on How to Look Skinny in a Photo [If You're Not Skinny].) These are the women who have the answers.

WE BELIEVE THAT YOUR VALUES ARE NOT OUR BUSINESS

We're not going to lecture you. Unlike other writers of diet books, we don't pretend to be your physician, your therapist, your shaman, or your mother. We won't tell you that in order to lose weight, you positively must transform your lifestyle, raise your self-esteem, keep a food journal, heal your soul, or find God. We are not going to push *sensible eating* down your throat. We're not going to force you to exercise. We won't even discuss your health. Most of our tips are quite healthy, but we will let you in on a few that are not. For instance, did you know that some women use Tylenol Sinus to speed up their metabolism? (See The Skinny on Speed [1].) That one woman we know pops a Valium and then turns on the TV whenever she is overcome with the desire to binge? Or that most women report that they lose a lot of weight whenever they go through extreme emotional turmoil? (See The Skinny on Misery, Anxiety, and Depression.) This doesn't mean we're promoting drugs or divorce—we're just stating the facts. We want you to know what REALLY WORKS. For us,

7

getting skinny is not about morality; it's about practicality.

Naturally, we will let you know the risks, but after that, the choice is yours. You're an adult. You know what your priorities are. If living is not one of them, go ahead and smoke. There's a good chance it will help you lose weight.

We Think It's Better to Have Lost and Gained Than Never Lost At All

The standard argument against diets is that they don't last, that the weight loss is temporary. An often-quoted government study claims that only one out of every two hundred people who try to lose weight succeeds in taking at least 10 pounds off and keeping them off for a year. So what? The benefits of a shower don't last either. You have to take one day after day after day for the rest of your life if you want to be clean. That doesn't mean you should throw up your hands and decide you might as well be dirty. The truth is that most diets work—that is, you will lose weight if you follow them. We realize, of course, it's not always so easy to stay on a diet. That is why we have provided strategies for motivating yourself to change your eating habits and then to stick with your new regimen.

"But no one can stay on a diet forever," the argument continues. Well, first of all, some people can and we have met them. But admittedly, most people do not spend a lifetime on a diet. They may diet serially, or they may give up forever. If they revert to their old eating and exercise habits, they will gain some weight back because sadly, a diet is not an immunization shot that protects you from gaining weight for the rest of your life. Contrary to popular belief, though, someone who goes off a diet will not in the long run necessarily gain MORE weight than she lost. Yo-yo dieting, many researchers now conclude, has no lasting effect, nor is it particularly harmful.

Anyway: Even if you do gain the weight back, wasn't it nice to have been skinny for a while?

We Don't Believe That Slow Is Necessarily Better

In some ways, it makes a lot of sense to go on a diet that promises to take off 10 pounds over ten years. At the end of ten years, after all, you will be 10 pounds thinner. But how boring! People who advocate moderate diets like this tell you that the weight you lose stays off longer than the weight you lose on wackier diets. Duh. You're on a diet longer!

We're not knocking the modest approach. It does work for a lot of people. It is less of a shock to the system, less drastic, and seems to target fat rather than muscle mass. However, there are some women who need the psychological boost of losing a significant amount of weight FAST in order then to diet more reasonably. "Oh, but that is only water weight," some people will object. Better to lose water weight than no weight at all, even if it returns. Besides, there are just some occasions where it behooves you to take off weight as fast as you can. If, for example, you must fit into your wedding gown next month, it's not a wise idea to reschedule the wedding for ten years later.

We Believe in Calories

We wish they didn't exist, but they do. And we think they are the key to a Skinny-shaping diet. In general, the more calories you eat, the more pounds you will gain. It doesn't matter if you eat them all at once, twelve times a day, late at night, or standing upside-down. We don't believe in negative-calories foods. We are also highly dubious about voodoo food combinations that somehow merge in your stomach to become more fattening than the calorie sum of their parts. And we have trouble with the concept of being allergic to certain foods in a way that makes you break out in fat (though indeed it may be that some types of food make you bloat).

But what about all those diets, like the Atkins' Diet, the Rice Diet, the many Low-Fat Diets, or the Ice-Cream Diet that allow you to eat unlimited amounts of calorie-rich foods? Well, a lot of those diets don't work for everyone. In the cases where they do—and we certainly have heard success stories—they seem to work by causing you to become satiated with high-calorie foods before you consume too many calories. In other words, it is a question of how many calories you eat before you get too sick to eat any more, no matter what kind of food you eat. (See The Skinny on Single-Food Diets.) If you can eat a cow every single day, you will gain weight, even though you had only protein.

Unfortunately, this does not mean that if you cut down your calorie intake by, say, 200 calories a day, you will continue to lose weight at the same rate you initially did. For when you lose weight, your metabolism—the rate at which your body converts fat into energy—eventually slows down. This is the bad news about dieting, not about losing weight by reducing your calories. Which brings us to another one of our convictions . . .

We Believe in Exercise, Too

Exercise seems to be the only non-pill way you can raise your metabolism. This does not mean that exercise alone will make you skinny; nor does it mean that you can eat whatever you want if you exercise. Being skinny is a function of both diet and exercise. We are concentrating on the former because there's just not a lot to say about exercise besides "Do it!" (For a discussion on how, when, and where to do it, see The Skinny on Exercise.) Moreover, as so many women told us, in the short run, you can lose weight by dieting without exercise, whereas it is far harder to lose weight by exercising alone. In the long run, you must do both.

That said, one item became clear during our Skinny Lunches: There are skinny people who never exercise and there are fat people who exercise fiendishly. We suspect that the skinnies are very active even if they don't go to a gym, and the fatties are using their workout as an excuse to overeat. But differences in preordained body chemistry cannot be overlooked. In other words . . .

We Believe That Life Is Not Fair

We saw a certain unnamed supermodel, whose weight is in the double digits, devour lamb chops, bread, and tiramisu in a New York restaurant. Of course, we later saw her in the ladies' room counteracting those calories, but that's another chapter. [See The Skinny on Speed (1)]. But even without chemical help, chances are that this unnamed model would have a thinner body than you. For one thing, metabolism is predetermined by and large. (Our apologies about the word choice.) You can change your metabolism fairly significantly through exercise, but 1) it's a lot of sustained work and 2) your body will still naturally gravitate to a certain weight. You were also genetically programmed to have a certain shape, which you can change to only a slight degree, unless you seek out the help of a plastic surgeon. (Sorry, but one only needs to look at tennis players to see that spot reducing is a myth. Though they exercise one arm predominantly, their fat content is fairly even distributed in both arms.) The shape you got is probably not your favorite shape in the world. What can you do? You can wear a sign that says *This Is Not the Way I Choose to Look,"* or you can rise above vanity and be happy whatever you weigh, or you can do all you can to fight against what we think of as the third law of thermodynamics: People tend to get fatter. You can still be skinny, but let's be real: Losing weight is not nearly as much fun as gaining weight. It's not fair, but it's true.

The Skinny On...
EATING DISORDERS

For a moment, we want to be utterly serious. We are aware of how devastating eating disorders can be, and we don't have any wish to encourage them. If you think your dieting habits are destructive or out of control, the advice in *The Skinny* isn't for you. If you have medical problems, *The Skinny* isn't for you. If you are a teenager, *The Skinny* isn't for you. It's for adults (we include ourselves in this category) who care about how they feel and look, but have a sane perspective about their health and well-being.

The Skinny

QUANTITY VS. QUALITY

A quantity eater enjoys the process of eating more than she enjoys the food itself. For her, "serving size" means the amount in the box or even the house. She tries to eat slowly—to drag out the experience—but often can't resist the impulse to eat fast. Taste is not as important as the sensation of putting edible stuff in her mouth. And not even always edible. She will eat grocery store brands, salad without dressing, even food that is a couple days past the expiration date if she's desperate. Just so she can keep eating. (What we mean by "she," of course, is "we.")

Quantity eaters, by the way, aren't the same as bingers: Bingers are sprinters; quantity eaters go for the distance. A quantity eater crunches on carrots all day long; the binger gobbles down a cake, a quart of ice cream, and a few loaves of bread in a matter of minutes and calls it a night. A capable quantity eater has enough stamina to turn a virtually zero-calorie food like lettuce into a source of weight gain. One Skinny Luncher told us that she became a vegetarian so she could eat for a longer amount of time with less chance of gaining weight.

A quality eater savors her food. She would rather not eat at all than eat inferior food. She is apt to be a food snob. She often prefers fattening food—rich sauces, fine pastries, greasy junk food. Yet, she rarely has a problem with her weight. She is satisfied with a bite, or at least a portion that is reasonably sized. Once she has tasted, she can stop—because the experience of eating is unimportant. The quality eater has no problem buying an ice-cream cone, taking a lick, and throwing the rest in the trash. She is lucky. We hate her.

If you are reading this book, you are probably a quantity eater. Or worse—a quantity quality eater—someone who likes vast amounts of choice food. Quality eaters think quantity eaters are either gluttons or mental cases who use food to redress some grave emotional need. They may be right, but then again, they may not. True, sometimes quantity eaters eat because they're bored or lonely or angry or depressed. But quality eaters skip meals for those very same reasons, so there goes that theory. Ultimately, nobody knows for sure what determines appetite.

But that doesn't stop scientists from having a lot of theories. The hypothalamus, a part of the brain, tells us when we're hungry, but unfortunately, it is not exactly clear what triggers the hypothalamus to go on or off. It seems we become hungry when the glucose levels in our body drop or when we have too few serotonin re-uptake inhibitors, too little adrenaline, or too many endorphines. Evolution is also blamed. For millions of years—before restaurants and convenience marts, buffets and takeout—food was scarce. Human beings consequently spent a lot of time foraging for food. In fact, there wasn't much else to do for fun. It was not only in our interest to accumulate as much food in the cave as possible, it was also a real plus to store gobs of body fat so that we could burn it during times of famine. Foods high in sugar and fat made us fattest and so we craved them most. Prehistoric cave drawings show cave men and women taking extreme measures to rob bees of their honey. Human beings, in other words, are hardwired to be fat.

Great! So you're a quantity eater but you want to be skinny. Now what do you do?

- Put nonfood things in your mouth. Chew on pencils. Bite your nails. Acquire a habit for drinking water and eating sawdust. Gnaw on the turkey bones instead of the turkey. Suck on a pacifier (in private). (See The Skinny on Sex.)
- Practice eating rituals that prolong or stop a meal. Notice that skinny people eat slowly. So should you. Cut up your food into ridiculously small pieces, then play with it on your plate. Chew your food until your jaw feels like it ran the marathon. Or better yet, suck on your food instead of chewing it. One woman told us she interrupts a meal by smoking a cigarette. Another told us she picks a fight with her husband, then leaves the dinner table in a huff. If you don't have a husband, go to a restaurant and become irked by the people at the table next to you. Which reminds us . . .
- Eat at restaurants where the service is slow as molasses (reduced-calorie molasses).
- Develop a disdain for your favorite fattening foods by overdosing. One woman told us she worked in an ice-cream parlor and will never eat ice cream again. Then she worked in a chocolate factory and will never eat chocolate again. Finally, she went to Japan and because she hates Japanese food, she ate

only Burger King for months. She will never step into a Burger King again. Okay, so maybe you don't have the time to work in an Entenmann's factory. You could at least devote an entire night to eating coffee cakes and hope to end up with a food aversion.

• Learn to have a contempt for cooking. Cook elaborate meals for your family for a month straight. Use the oven a lot in the summer in a kitchen without air-conditioning. Make your own condiments.

The Skinny

MAKING IT LOOK BIG

A skinny man we know told us that he is a closet dieter, his favorite regimen being eight consecutive meals of total deprivation followed by one All-You-Want-of-Anything Feast. The last part is easy, but how does he survive the lean times? Among his tips are methods for making small amounts of foods look like large amounts of food—and all without mirrors and magnifying glasses. Mr. Skinny adds water to eggs before he scrambles them, puts anything he can in a blender with ice, and dices fruit rather than eating it whole. (He claims he can cut a large naval orange into 30 or 40 chunks in under a minute.) Eating apple slices with a fork, he says, adds to the illusion that you are having a lavish meal and not a snack. Using his Silo Technique, he stacks his food—say, broccoli or salad nicoise—adding extra height by placing the heap on a bed of lettuce or dry rice. (We imagine Styrofoam packing pellets would work, too.) Tall and thin, he says, is better than short and wide. As short women, we'd like to object. Short food can seem substantial, too. Think of carpaccio—mere specks of meat or fish flattened to such a degree that it can cover an area as large as Texas and take as long to eat as a drive through that state.

The Skinny

CALORIES PER MINUTE

Sure calories matter, but they're only part of the formula. What also has to be taken into consideration is how many calories you're eating per minute, in other words, the *rate* of calorie consumption. Slow Food, the slower the better, is the key to weight loss.

What's Slow Food? Well, you've heard of Fast Food, right? Fast food is convenient, cheap, and plentiful. It tends to be dense in calories and easy to eat, a deadly combination. In less time than it takes to say *"Double Whopper,"* you can eat approximately a million calories worth of fast food. Not so with Slow Food. Between the time you think about eating Slow Food and the time you actually put it in your mouth, a long, long time can elapse. You can wither away. This is because Slow Food is often hard to find (for instance, mamey colorados, a fruit found only in the hinterlands of Cuba), hard to prepare (for instance, mussels, which must be scrubbed for hours before they can be cooked), or—as is just about always the case—hard to eat. Slow Food is so hard to eat, you often give up before you finish. Whether Slow Food is high or low in calories per serving is not its most defining characteristic. What is most important is that it is low in *Calories Per Minute*.

Let's compare, for instance, dry roasted cashews and pistachios. Both are high in calories—about 160 calories an ounce. Pistachios in their shells, however, are much lower in calories per minute (CPM) than cashews because of the time spent prying them open. Specifically: One ounce of dry roasted cashews, about 18 medium nuts, is 163 calories. Based on an informal survey, we determined that the average person eats about 20 cashews per minute. Cashews, therefore, have 181 calories per minute (CPM). An ounce of dry roasted pistachios with shells, about 25 nuts, is 160 calories. The average person, however, can shell and eat only 8 pistachio nuts per minute. The CPM of pistachios, then, is 51. The difference in calories per ounce is marginal, but the pistachios with shells are unquestionably the Skinny Choice. (The CPM for pistachios can be even lower than 80 because you are likely to get stuck on a particularly hard-to-crack nut or even break your nail and have to stop eating nuts for a while. If you are very lucky, you will slice open your finger on a shell and have to go to the hospital, where you will cause the CPM to go down even farther. We advise, therefore, to buy the pistachio nuts that must be opened with power tools.)

There are tricks to lowering the CPM of a food. For instance, take cereal. It takes no time to eat a bowl or two or three or four of cereal. However, if the cereal is Raisin Bran and you hate raisins, it could take hours to get through a couple bowls. Now, eat the cereal with a baby spoon. . . .

FOODS NATURALLY LOW IN CPM

FOOD	CALORIES/MINUTES	CPM
1-lb lobster (steamed; no butter unless you spill it)	95 cal/ 25 minutes	3.8
4-oz crab (steamed)	110 cal/9 minutes	12.2
Escargot in garlic butter sauce	30 cal/2 minutes	15
9.7-oz pomegranate	104 cal/16 minutes	6.5
1 large artichoke	23 cal/10 minutes	2.3
1 slice, 10-in. diameter watermelon (includes taking seeds out before each bite)	152 cal/4 minutes	38
3³/₄-oz can sardines in oil, drained	130 cal/impossible to open	0

The Skinny

EATING PEANUTS

No.*

*32 cups of air-popped popcorn without butter = 1 cup of peanuts.

The Skinny

THE FDA

Have you ever had the sneaking suspicion that the Food and Drug Administration (the FDA) lies? That they have a secret plan to make you fat by telling you that cottage cheese is 22 calories per tablespoon when in fact it is 220? Don't worry: To the best of their knowledge, the information printed on food labels is truthful. However—and here's where you can really be paranoid—the FDA's source is none other than the food companies. The police ask the criminal for a report of the crime?! Okay, calm down. The FDA randomly tests hundreds of products to verify accuracy. However—paranoia alert!—as of August 1998, they had conducted periodic testing only twice since 1993. Hold on, don't jump! If you suggest to the FDA that a company might be lying about their calorie count, the FDA will reanalyze the product.

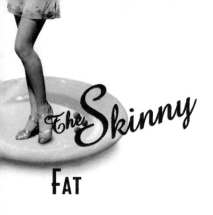

FAT

Fat is a richly nuanced, densely metaphorical word. You are fat, you have fat, you eat fat, you are fat-free, fat is you. *Le fat, c'est moi.* Let us differentiate and define each layer of fatness.

1. You Are Fat

You are obese, corpulent, fleshy, overblown, plump, ripe, chubby, portly, stout, stocky, beefy, ample, more-than-ample, burly, pudgy, tubby, heavy, thickset, round, blobby, big, big-boned, hefty, chunky, dumpy, rotund. Your clothes don't fit. You are fat.

2. You Have Fat

The average person has anywhere from twelve to thirty pounds of body fat, which is stored in your liver, around your internal organs, under your skin, and on that part of your thigh that your favorite skirt, unfortunately, exposes. A pound of body fat has about 3,500 calories, so the average person's body fat is roughly 42,000 to 105,000 calories. Most people have enough body fat to live without food for sixty days.

Your body stores fat in special "fat cells" and burns it for energy. These fat cells are formed all the time, but most of them are created at specific times in your life: In the final month or so before you're born, in your first two years of life, and in the last two years before you enter puberty. The really depressing news is that apparently, fat cells never die. They shrink, they shrivel, but they never disappear entirely, except through liposuction. If you lose weight, your fat cells get emptied out, but the cell itself remains and can be refilled anytime you decide to eat cheesecake. If you were fat as a kid (or an embryo, actually) you probably have more fat cells than someone who does their ballooning a little later in life. This doesn't mean you can't get thin; it just means that you have more little cellular pockets just dying to fill up with extra calories. If you weren't fat as a kid, don't get too cocky: Your body will build more fat cells if you insist on having a quart of Rocky Road ice cream every night and your existing cells just aren't roomy enough for all your blubber.

By the way, fat cells store extra calories from any food source, not just extra calories from ingested fat. Your body is perfectly programmed to convert any and all food products to fat. Sirloin steaks, salad dressing, Boston cream pie, tofu, whatever: If you eat too much, it will be stashed away for future self-abuse in your body-fat cells.

Measuring your body fat tells you how much of your total weight is made up of, well, blubber, versus bones, muscles, fluids, and organs. The generally accepted ideal body-fat percentages are 15–25 percent for women and 5–15 percent for men. You can gauge body fat by bioelectrical impedance (an electric current is sent through your body—painlessly, of course—and measured); by skinfold dimensions (a caliper measures fat pinched at four different body sites); by anthropometric measurements (calculations are based on the circumference measurements of your stomach, thigh, and calf). It's worth knowing what your body fat is so that you can brag about it and also so that you can see whether you're losing fat off of your body or just water or muscle. Also, if you're exercising and dieting, your weight might not change that much because you'll be building muscles, which weigh a lot, but your body composition might have changed considerably, and that's worth knowing. In a way, this is not that much different from assessing your weight by using a pair of pants rather than a scale, because it shows how much space your body is occupying, which we believe is much more important than the numbers on a scale. Once you decide you want to measure your fat, here are your choices. You can buy a bioelectrical impedance scale—they're about $150 dollars and not much bigger than a household scale (call 1-800-982-6482 for information on Tanita BIA scales; otherwise ask at a medical-supply or fitness store or a weight-loss center). Or you can buy calipers and measure your own skinfolds—calipers are pretty cheap—although the chance that you'll not measure the same exact places each time means your results might vary like crazy. If you're still sold on the caliper idea, see if your gym or doctor does a skinfold measurement. They are more likely to be consistent at it, although we personally have had caliper tests that have varied by as much as 10 percent. That's scary.

For the anthropometrically minded, there's a free Internet service that will calculate your body fat based on your tape-measure results, www.biofitness.com/abodyfat.html. And by the way, you can also just keep a comparative record of those abdomen/thigh/calf inches on your own; it won't give you percentages, but it will be a good indicator of whether you're growing or shrinking in stature.

3. You Eat Fat

And how! There's fat in almost everything, from olives to ostrich steaks to (in trace amounts) oatmeal. This is important because of simple mathematics: Fat in food has 9 calories per gram, while carbohydrates and protein have about 4.5 calories per gram. Plus, fat is nice and compact. One tablespoon of cooking oil has 128 calories. Twelve cups of endive has 120 calories. About eight ounces of cod has 160 calories. In other words, you get a lot more bang for your buck, quantity-wise, with carbohydrates and proteins than with fat.

On top of that, your body can process fat so easily that you lose only 6 percent of those calories in the digesting of them, while burning up twelve cups of endive would use up 15 percent of the calories, and burning eight ounces of cod would use 25 percent of its caloric value. Which means that the real, post-digestion cost of these three foods is:

Tablespoon of cooking oil (128 minus 6 percent) = 120.32 calories

Twelve cups of endive (120 minus 15 percent) = 102 calories

Eight-ounce portion of cod (160 minus 25 percent) = 120 calories

Which means, essentially, that fat is more fattening than other foods. Which is actually great news, because it means that if you limit your consumption of fat, you will automatically be cutting your calories without necessarily noticing a dramatic decrease in your food. If you have a bialy for breakfast instead of a blueberry muffin, it won't necessarily feel that different. But, because the bialy has almost no fat and a muffin can have as many as 26 grams (Sara Lee, large corn muffin) the difference in calories is astonishing: 300 for the bialy versus 490 for the muffin.

You do need to eat a certain amount of fat to do little things like keeping your reproductive system operating, preserving brain function, maintaining your body temperature at 98.6. If you eat any meat or any eggs, you are getting some fat; there's also a lot of fat in some surprising places, like in avocados, salmon, and biscotti. Our personal theory is that you should always opt for anything you can eat fat-free that doesn't seem any the worse for it—yogurt, milk, breakfast cereal, and crackers for instance; you should also pick low-fat meats like chicken over high-fat meats like filet mignons; you should also go for fish instead of land animals whenever you can, because it is almost always lower in fat.

Go ahead: Cite all those annoying facts about people in Burgundy, France, who live on foie gras and almonds and are still twiggy. Our attitude? Good for them and we just don't believe it. They don't call it fat for nothing, sister.

4. You Are Fat-Free

Not so fast. Low-fat or fat-free diets are NOT calorie-free; they're just reduced in a way that is not so horribly painful (isn't it easier to skip the butter than the bread?). The trouble is if you eat huge amounts of fat-free things, you will get fat! Because once again, you're eating too many calories! And this is also why it has been demonstrated that Americans are eating less fat than ever but are fatter than ever. A paradox, yes, but completely understandable, as anyone who has eaten a whole box of Snackwells at one sitting can attest. Fat-free living is not a goal in itself—it's a method for cutting down on calories so you will lose weight. We used to go jogging with a very stout woman who complained that she was running five miles a day and wasn't losing any weight even though she was eating nothing but bagels. "They're fat-free!" she declared, jiggling in her Nikes. "I don't get it!" We do. A bagel has almost no fat, but depending on its size, it can have as many as 600 calories. If you run five miles, you haven't even burned up one big bagel's worth of energy. Don't be discouraged. Just don't be fooled. A pint of fat-free frozen yogurt is better than a pint of super-rich ice cream, but it's still dessert.

The Skinny

THE BEST WAY TO LOOK SKINNY

Hang out with fat people.

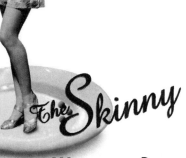

What to Do if You Really, Really Need to Lose Five Pounds in Five Minutes

Sometimes (maybe lots of times, actually) you will find yourself in a Code Red situation—that is, you have an upcoming wedding/graduation/job interview/photo session/important party/blind date/class reunion/new, expensive, slightly-too-tight dress that you can't return/first encounter with an old boyfriend/appearance before the Supreme Court—and you really, really have to look skinnier fast. In situations like these, "moderation" is a curse word. You don't have time for anything, let alone for being sensible. We can't help you if you're trying to go from a size 14 plus to a 4 petite in time for your appearance on CNN tomorrow, but here's what to do if you need to get as lean as you can as fast as you can:

If You Have One Day to Lose

You've been merrily stuffing your face all weekend and suddenly remember that on Tuesday you're going to the White House for dinner and the dress you're planning to wear will cause your lungs to collapse if you aren't just the right size:

1. Call a good dressmaker—just in case.
2. Immediately drink a lot of water—not that it helps you lose weight, but it makes you think you're going to, which helps.
3. We advocate fasting, although there are people (scientists, actually) who say that there is no real difference between eating nothing for a day and eating 800 calories, so you might rather opt for the 800.
4. In which case, eat 800 calories of lean protein, no carbohydrates, no fat. That could be 800 calories of turkey breast, water-packed tuna, egg whites, or perhaps an 800-calorie turkey/tuna/egg white omelet, if you insist.
5. Keep drinking lots of water and tea. You really will feel virtuous.
6. Don't take any ibuprofen. Why? Because we once heard an interview with Ice, one of those scary-looking women on *American Gladiators* who has way too many muscles but has absolutely no flab anywhere on her rock-hard body, and she said that before photo shoots she never takes ibuprofen because it makes her bloat. We're sure she's too modest to tell us where she received her Ph.D. in biophysics, but she most certainly has one, don't you think? So we live by her advice on this one.

IF YOU HAVE ONE WEEK TO LOSE

1. Do everything we just said, *plus*
2. Maybe you can't stick to the 800-calorie diet, and you probably shouldn't. Instead, you can add a few calories but stay on the protein side of the road.

3. Our friend Gully Wells, an editor at Conde Nast *Traveler,* advocates the Sashimi-Espresso-Nicotine diet for crisis management. You get your protein (sashimi), your boost-cum-dessert (espresso), and your oral-cravings pacifier (Marlboro Lights). You can probably also do this without the Marlboro Lights, too.

4. Don't exercise like a maniac. It'll only make you hungry and self-pitying. On the other hand, stay active. Then try to schedule at least one session of some kind of exercise which you will do for over an hour. Even if it's walking, try to keep yourself working at something for an hour. If you can do it more than once in the week, that's even better. The reason for this is your body seems to really get metabolically super-charged once you get it going for more than an hour—it's a trick marathon runners do in order to deplete as much of their stored glycogen as possible before they carbo-load for the race. Therefore, deplete your glycogen and skip the carbo-loading and you will end up leaner.

5. Eat lots of parsley. It's a natural diuretic. It also has a lot of vitamins, which is valuable if you're not eating much food.

6. Consume vinegar. We don't know why, but a lot of people at our Skinny Lunches swore that vinegar helped them pare down. Some put a teaspoon in water and drank it, some doused their parsley salad with it, some added it to their omelets. . . . Some even guzzled it from the bottle (3 T. a day). Whether vinegar's slimming powers are a myth or not, we can't say, but why not try it?

7. Wear your most urchinlike clothes. We find that catching glimpses of ourselves looking waifish (or as waifish as one can look if one is in fact portly) actually spurs us on to victory. We see ourselves and think, *Look how frail and delicate I am! A person like me must eat like a bird!*

   However, if you're one of those people who looks at herself in the mirror and thinks, *Oh. My. God. I look peaked, I should eat something,* then don't look in any mirrors this week. Also, you might want to reference this reaction when you're trying to figure out why you weigh too much.

8. At least for this week, everything counts. Free samples, cream in your coffee, chewing gum— most of the time you can overlook a lot of these trifles, but when you're on a mission you have to be tough. Stick to your guns.

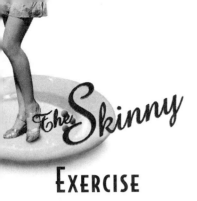

The Skinny

EXERCISE

Here it is: The chapter you always skip in diet books! And who can blame you? After all, who doesn't know by now (and feel guilty about the fact) that 1) we need to exercise and 2) we don't get enough exercise. Remember what we told you about exercise?

We repeat: Exercise matters. A few women at the Skinny Lunches declared themselves exercise-free, but our guess is that they are magical creatures who eat air and dissolve in rainstorms. Also, we don't believe them. Perhaps they are not gym regulars, but they probably walk and fidget more than they realize, or more likely they're lying in order to preserve the image of effortless elegance and slimness while in fact they run eight miles a day. Since we and most women we know do not have one of those combustible metabolisms and aren't good at lying, we have to be practical. Therefore, we endorse exercise as a diet tool. Our idea of exercise is not an Olympian regime or a body-building program that will land you in an abs-of-platinum competition—we simply advise a certain steady amount of activity because it will help you lose weight and not gain it back. Coincidentally, regular exercise will also make you healthier as well as skinnier, but that's not our fault. We are for the moment only interested in exercise as a weight-loss technique (tips about heart disease, antioxidants, or VO_{2Max} rates we'll save for our next book, *The Flabby*).

SEVERAL REASONS WHY EXERCISE IS A GOOD IDEA FOR ANYONE INTERESTED IN BECOMING SKINNY

1. It burns calories.
2. It burns calories.
3. It burns calories.
4. Only very, very skillful people can eat while exercising, so a significant benefit of exercise is that the more time you spend doing it, the less time you will have for eating. Also, most people find it unpleasant to eat right before they exercise, so if you have a regular workout schedule, that preexercise no-eating time should add another hour or so of noneating to your day. Also, if you exercise when you're hungry, you will forget that you're hungry, or at least you will delay eating because you're busy exercising, and by the time you're done exercising, you're so preoccupied with being tired, sweaty, sore, etc., that you will forget that you were starving.
5. It is so crushingly depressing to look fat in exercise clothes that if you start working out you will be even more motivated to get thin.
6. People who claim that exercise makes them hungry are just plain wrong. Scientifically speaking, sustained activity increases your body's production of noradrenaline, a hormone that is a natural appetite suppressant. Intense exercise can increase your body's nonadrena-

line to as much as five times normal levels, and the appetite-suppressing effects can last for as long as six or eight hours after exercise. Being ravenously hungry after exercising is all in your mind. What this means is that gorging on a dozen bagels after running a mile is a choice (a bad choice), not an imperative.

7. If you diet but don't exercise, you can lose weight. However, the weight you lose from dieting alone will consist of water, fat, and as much as fifty percent lean muscle. If you diet plus you exercise, the weight you will lose will consist of water, some muscle, but more fat than if you were only dieting. It is better to lose fat than muscle. A pound of muscle burns more calories than a pound of fat all the time, just to sustain itself, so if your body has more muscles you will burn more calories all the time, exercising or not. Muscles are good. They do not have to be big and bulgy to be metabolically useful (think of ballerinas—pure muscle and oh so skinny). What you want, ideally, is to have a body that is the size and shape you want, but is made up of muscles rather than fat, because your metabolism will be higher and it will be harder for you to gain weight. A lean, lithe, muscular size 6 person can use up as many as 800 more calories a day just being alive than a blubbery size 6 person does.

8. One little underappreciated benefit of exercise is that it makes you arrogant. There's nothing quite as satisfying as Rollerblading past someone who is sitting on a park bench eating

Doritos. This means the next time you have a choice between your very own bag of Doritos and going Rollerblading, you will be more likely to choose the Rollerblades. Adopting an athlete's fascistic, contemptuous *Ubermensch* attitude (*my body is a sacred and well-tooled superior machine, maybe I should skip the mayonnaise,* blah blah blah) is not a bad state of mind when you're trying to lose weight.

9. Exercise gets easier as you weigh less, which means that the more you work out the easier it will feel, which in turn makes it more appealing to work out. And so forth.

10. If you believe in the concept of a "setpoint"—a weight that your body naturally gravitates toward—be aware that scientists think the only permanent way to change that setpoint is through exercise, because it changes your muscle/fat ratio which increases the calories you need each day to stay alive.

WHICH EXERCISES MAKE YOU SKINNY?

The only exercise that will make you skinny is exercise you will actually, seriously, honestly, consistently do. Don't say you're going to train for the marathon if you secretly hate to run, and don't commit to playing tennis five times a week if you don't have a partner—settle on something you like (or like well enough, if you hate any form of activity) and something you have time for and can accomplish easily. If you want to exercise by doing a few things rather than just one, be sure to make a schedule for yourself. If you want to bike two days a week and swim three, then pick those days in advance and plan on it. For that matter, make a schedule for yourself no matter what. Studies show that people who have an exercise routine stick with it far longer than people who don't.

You should probably start by considering how much time you can spend working out. For the sake of comparison, here are the calories burned in a half hour by different forms of exercise:

Lying down motionlessly	45
Walking	100
Swimming	300
Stationary bicycle	150
Moving bicycle	175
Running, nine-minute pace	360
Rowing	175
Ice skating	225
Roller skating	225
Energetic dancing	250
Jumping rope	400
Cross-country skiing	275
Racquetball, squash	450
Tennis	150

Most people with real lives, jobs, friends, errands, families, and so forth, do not have unlimited amounts of time to exercise, so the efficiency of your workout makes a big difference in how skinny it will help you become. Case in point: Moving yourself for a mile on foot burns about 100 calories, whether you walk, hop, or run the mile at a marathon pace. If you walk a mile, it takes about twenty minutes. If you run at an average speed, you can cover a mile in about ten minutes. If you have allotted, say, forty minutes for exercise, you can either:

—Walk two miles and burn 200 calories, or

—Run four miles and burn 400 calories, or

—Run really fast and cover about six miles and use up 600 calories.

You could, of course, walk six miles and burn the same 600 calories, but walking will take you about two hours. Walking for weight loss really works only for people who have a lot of spare time or who can incorporate it into their daily routine as transportation. That is, if you live two miles from your office and can walk there and back every day, you can write it off as exercise and not lift another finger. Again, it's a matter of time. If you can play tennis for hours and hours a day, lucky you; otherwise, the intensity of squash and racquetball make them much more effective if you want to burn calories and lose weight and you only have a normal forty- or fifty-minute exercise slot in your life.

Some forms of exercise are very intense but hard to sustain. Jumping rope, for instance, burns calories like crazy, but it is very hard to jump for long enough to burn off the equivalent of a chocolate-chip cookie. On the other hand, if you can build up the strength to jump rope for ten minutes straight or more, it will burn as many calories per minute as running at a seven-minute-per-mile pace, which is nice and speedy. If you can build up to jumping rope for forty minutes, you have our undying admiration and also you're probably cheating. If you're not, you will be using up about 600 calories in forty minutes, which is about as good as it gets.

The harder a physical activity feels, the more calories it probably burns. If it feels easy, it probably is.

You can make up for easiness by doing the easy thing for a longer amount of time and end up burning plenty of calories. Realistically, though, the best way to exercise is to get good enough at an activity to do it pretty intensely, and to get strong enough to do it for a decent period of time, and to like it enough that you can get yourself to do it several times a week.

How Many Times a Week, Really?

Anything is better than nothing; three times a week is good; five times a week is very, very good. Believe it or not, it's easier to exercise at least three times a week because you get used to doing it and it becomes less of an ordeal each time. One maniac we know (with a great body) runs every single day because she says she can't stand deciding about whether or not she feels like running; she just does it automatically and eliminates the temptation to put it off for another day. This is not a recommendation—it's just an observation. For more moderate people, working out every other day would be a good schedule. Or just working out on weekdays. The important thing to realize is that you won't really see the effects of exercise until you're at it three times a week or more. Working out less often than that isn't useless, but it won't necessarily make you feel that much different.

How Long Do I Have to Punish Myself?

The gold standard for exercise is forty minutes, because your body shifts from burning carbohydrates to burning fats at that point, and it's nice to use up fat. On the other hand, even a little bit of exercise is worth doing, and we've read several recent studies that suggest that the "burning carbohydrate vs. burning fat" rule is mostly myth: Burning calories is burning calories, wherever they come from. One recent report says that working out several times a day for ten minutes each time is really just as good as working out for one long stretch; it's just inconvenient if you end up having to shower four times a day. If you want to see yourself wasting away into something gorgeous and svelte, you really should get in around four hours of exercise a week, divided up whichever way you want. Two things to remember: If you are only going to work out for a short time, make it a hard short time—it's a lot more shrewd to run for fifteen minutes than to walk for fifteen minutes, because you'll use so many more calories. And if you can exercise once a week for a long time—ideally an hour—you will get a bonus calorie-burn (somehow your body goes into overdrive if you push it for a long time once a week or so).

Okay, I'm Going to Try to Work Out Three or Four Times a Week for About Forty Minutes or So. What Should I Do?

Here are our personal recommendations for exercise:

—RUNNING. If you can take the banging and jostling, running is one of the best possible ways to work out for skinniness. It burns tons of calories, quickly. It doesn't build up any weird, bulky muscles. It's easy to do once you build up your strength. It can be done pretty much anywhere. If you happen to travel a lot, it's very transportable. It's cheap. It can be done with people or alone. It's completely adjustable—that is, if you have only twenty minutes, you can go out and sprint hard and make it worthwhile; if you have an hour, you can be leisurely and get a lot of benefits.

The downside to running: Running is hard on your body, so you're likely to have injuries now and then. There are also some horrifying warnings being issued that it might break down the collagen in your face (all that bouncing, we guess) which would result in a very saggy profile, but we'll keep running until that's a proven fact and anyway, isn't that what facelifts are for? Also, if you're a wimp about weather, you have to make sure you have access to a treadmill or be serious about an alternative when you think it's too cold/hot/humid/windy/rainy to go outside. It can get boring if you run alone or don't listen to music. Running makes your feet really ugly and gnarly. It's easy to get lazy and run too slow or not long enough to make it worthwhile.

How to run yourself skinny: Before you begin, go to a sporting-goods store (preferably one that specializes in running) and get fitted for good running shoes. You will be amazed at how much more pleasant it is to run with shoes that fit right. This is really, really crucial. Running with a partner or a group makes a huge difference; motivational psychologists who study these things say that people who exercise with a partner stick to it longer and more enthusiastically than solos. If you can't find anyone to run with you and can't afford to pay for a trainer to go with you, do your run somewhere popular and try to tag alongside someone who is going your speed—even that helps keep you going. Find out if there are any running groups in your area; even if you join them only once a week, you'll be amazed at how much it motivates you to be in a pack.

Buy yourself a Walkman or a portable CD player. It does look dorky to run with headphones, but people who work out to music can go up to 20 percent longer than people who don't (this is a scientific fact, by the way). Keeping a daily log also seems to help keep you motivated. (What is it about logs, anyway? Apparently keeping a log of what you eat helps motivate you, too.) There are road races everywhere these days. Even if you do not think of yourself as a racer, pick one as a goal for yourself, even if you just plan to walk it. This works because having a specific mission helps keep you going.

If you've never run before or are hopelessly out of shape and wheezy, start slowly. One good technique is to jog a minute, then walk a minute, and repeat for twenty minutes. Over the next few days/weeks, start jogging more and walking less. When you're starting out, it's better to keep track of how long you've run than how far you've run. Once you are able to run for forty minutes (even if it's at a very slow pace) you can start thinking in miles.

If you can run forty minutes three times a week, you will lose weight. This is virtually guaranteed, unless you end your runs at a Dunkin' Donuts. Once you can go forty minutes slowly, try to run a little faster for forty minutes. You will lose more weight.

—SQUASH OR RACQUETBALL. Both are great for those aspiring to skinniness because they burn so many calories. Both sports are simple to learn and play sort of decently—that is, decently enough to burn a lot of calories. Also, it's fairly easy to stay inspired because you're playing games with skills and scores and all that vicious competitive stuff that makes life interesting. Also, unless you're amoral, you will feel too guilty to bail out on your partner just because you feel lazy, so you'll stick to a schedule without even realizing it.

Downside: Requires a partner(s) and a court. Hard to keep on a routine if you travel or have an erratic work schedule. Sounds incredibly preppy (you might consider this a plus rather than a minus, of course).

How to make squash yourself skinny: Join a racquet club, invest in a few lessons, and then ask the pro to help you find partners. Or join a league so you have regular games. Most people will probably find it hard to get four or five games organized a week, so it's best to consider it as a secondary exercise—for instance, replace one or two running/workout days with games.

—IN-LINE SKATING. Rollerblading definitely burns calories and works your muscles, if you can learn to do it without killing yourself and have access to a good place to skate. If you can skate for transportation, you will be solving the time problem (that is, the I-don't-want-to-waste-time-exercising problem) and the burning-calories problem simultaneously. It's easier on your knees and ankles than running, and burns more calories than bicycling.

Downside: It's not for nothing that emergency-room doctors call Rollerblades "donor blades"—in-line skating is, no kidding, dangerous, not just because you'll strain hamstrings or pull muscles but because you might possibly kill yourself, either by falling on your head or running into an immovable object or by being hit by a movable object, i.e., an automobile, bicycle, or other Rollerblader. Also, it's easy to cheat—glide, go downhill, coast—so you might go out for an hour and really only burn up a handful of calories. It's also hard to skate at night and in bad weather.

How to skate to slenderness: Find somewhere you can skate hard, for real, for a set amount of time, or figure out how to skate to and from somewhere (your Weight Watchers meeting, perhaps?) regularly. If you skate for an hour and you don't feel tired, you're not skating hard enough, so either go faster or find somewhere that's more challenging for your workout. Hills are good—uphill, that is.

—GYMS. Ugh. Still and all, working out in a gym is a reliable way to burn up energy and whittle yourself into fabulous slenderness or something like that. Any idiot can use the equipment, and if you don't screw around you can work out effectively in a fixed amount of time. There are no environmental obstacles (as in: rain, heat, light) and what with all the television sets, video displays, new machines, and junky magazines to read while you're struggling along, going to the gym can be almost bearable.

Downside: We said "almost bearable," didn't we? What could be more horrible than forty minutes pedaling to nowhere or rowing into infinity? What could smell worse than a gym on a hot day? What sound could be more numbing than the grind of an unlubricated Precor Gym Trainer over the blare of MSNBC?

How to get gym-thin: If you have forty-five minutes to spend in the gym, focus on the treadmill, the cross-country ski machine, the Versa Climber, the rowing machine, or the stationary bike. StairMasters are okay but if you lean on the bars at all you are getting almost no benefit out of the workout—that is why people can do the StairMaster for hours at a time! Because it's not that hard if you're leaning on the armrests! (Also, anecdotal evidence suggests that StairMastering gives you a big butt.) Some people find it easiest to zone out for forty-five minutes on one machine, but if you get too restless (or your gym is crowded and has time limits), try doing a circuit of ten minutes on each of four machines—sometimes the time will go much faster that way. If you go to the gym with a friend, be serious and figure out how much time you're really working hard and how much time you're wasting. If, for instance, you find that you don't even need a shower after an hour at the gym with a friend, you're probably not working hard. We, personally, hate gyms, but we use them when necessary, and even though we're jealous when we see happy pairs of friends chatting away on tandem rowing machines, we tend to prefer going alone, grinding through our requisite minutes, and getting the hell out. Doing the weight machines is a whole different issue. You burn only about 300 calories an hour lifting weights (or using Nautilus-type equipment) so it isn't a big calorie-user; in fact, you could burn more calories walking for an hour. Nevertheless, there is one school of thought that says that building up your muscles is crucial, even if it doesn't burn calories, because it gives you more of that lean muscle mass that you need to perk up your metabolism. Timewise, if we have to choose between aerobic exercise and weight training, we always go for the aerobic stuff, because it makes us feel happier and thinner. Also we have an irrational fear of developing giant ropey muscles (we say "irrational" because unless you take steroids, you're not going to develop giant ropey muscles, and if you ever saw us doing the lateral lift Nautilus you'd really know that we're never going to develop giant ropey muscles). But if you've ever seen that little indent in your bicep because the muscle is getting larger and the fat is shrinking, then you know how much fun building a few select muscles can be, so if you've got time, do something that makes you sweat and then twice a week lift a dumbbell.

—SWIMMING. People claim that you can get thin from swimming, and it does have the advantage of being pretty much pain-free, as exercise goes. It's hard to hurt yourself unless you dive headfirst into the shallow end, and you never get hot, plus swimming doesn't destroy your knees and ankles. Also, some people think that you burn extra calories when you're swimming because you're cold and your body has to work to keep itself at 98.6 degrees (maybe, but our sources say the extra calories are negligible).

Downside: Quite honestly, are the people whose bodies you admire at the beach ever the ones who are in the water? We bet not. We bet the bodies you admire are sprawled prone on the chaise lounge, drinking diet Cokes. The problem with swimming is it's hard to do it long enough and vigorously enough to really get a calorie burn. You can't dog-paddle for twenty minutes and consider yourself slimmed; you have to swim hard for a real distance, which takes real time, and most people don't do that. Also, call us crazy, but aren't you always ravenously, uncontrollably hungry after you've been in the water?

How to swim slim: It seems like the only way you can make swimming work is if you have a coach or a team that can keep you honest as far as how fast and how long you swim. Or if you have a buddy who is willing to swim with you—but it has to be a buddy who is unyielding, punitive, critical, and slavedriving, because otherwise, girlfriends, you're going to be wasting your time. See, our assumption is that all is entropy, and that a body not forced to exercise will go buy an ice-cream cone, so if you don't put yourself in a position where you must exercise, you won't. It's just too easy to float rather than swim hard, so we're leery. If you love the water, then swim, but if you don't feel crummy when you're done with a session, you haven't been swimming hard enough to make it worth your time. In which case, put on your tennis shoes and walk up a twenty-story building.

—BICYCLING. Ditto everything said previously about Rollerblading. Biking is great exercise but only if you go for long, hard distances and add into the calculation how much time you spend coasting.

Downside: Not too many to speak of, except for those dorky bicycle clothes people seem compelled to wear. Also, bicycling does build up your thighs, which is probably the one part of our bodies that we never, ever think needs building up.

How to bike yourself skinny: When we bicycle, we consider the time we spend, not the mileage; in other words, if we bicycle five miles and it takes us twenty minutes, we don't think of it the same way as walking or running five miles, we think of it as twenty minutes of exercise, which converts to only about two miles of running. This keeps you honest. We also suggest you use a clunky, simple bicycle rather than one with a million speeds and plutonium frames—the heavier the bike and the harder it is to ride, the more calories you'll be burning. Most important, though, you've just got to ride for a long, long time to get slim. Ten minutes on flat ground and no sweating is not the way to slenderness. A good program is to run or go to the gym during the week and go on a long, long bike ride on the weekend.

Obviously, there are dozens of other ways to work out. The important issues are 1) that you do something and 2) that you aren't cheating, because if you're going to waste your time you might as well not bother exercising and instead do something really productive like cleaning your closets. Also, the worst thing about doing a cheater's workout is that sometimes exercising will make you feel so good and so powerful and so drained of calories that you will celebrate by eating a lot. If you have really burned up some pounds, it's not that bad to treat yourself, but if you inhale a bag of Pepperidge Farm cookies because you just did an hour on the StairMaster but were leaning on the bars the whole time and burned a total of four calories, you're going to get fat. Sorry.

While we're going negative, we might as well address the useless-exercise issue. There are plenty of workouts that have attained legendary weight-loss status but don't work, and as sad as it may be, it's better to know it now than to do them and be discouraged because you aren't losing an ounce:

1. **Anything having to do with heat (heat belts, sauna, rubber or nylon sweat suits, body wraps).**

Sweating because you're hot is not the same as sweating because you're mountain-climbing. If it were the same, why isn't everyone in Florida skinny?

2. Golf. Except if you're a caddy.

3. Spot-reducing exercises. You will lose fat from wherever your body chooses to lose it, no matter what. If you're exercising and creating an energy deficit, your metabolism will scoop up fuel from anywhere it locates it, not from the area that you're exercising. Yes, doing sit-ups flattens your stomach because it makes your stomach muscles strong and because you are using up energy, not because the sit-ups are actually burning the fat on your stomach. The rule of thumb (or thigh, as the case may be) is that you lose it first where it is stored last, so if you think about the way your body changes when you're chubby and just reverse that order, you'll have a pretty good idea of what will happen when you start losing weight. If you first balloon around your waist, then your rear end, then your upper arms, and lastly your neck and jowls, you will lose by first shrinking in your neck and jowls, then upper arms, then rear, and last, your waist. Since the oldest fat places on you are probably the ones you hate the most—familiarity breeding contempt—you'll have to be patient, since that's probably going to be the last fat you lose. On the other hand, people who complain that no matter how much weight they lose they never have a skinny whatever (butt, let's say) just haven't lost enough weight yet.

4. Sex. It is true that vigorous and sustained intercourse can use up 250 calories an hour, but when was the last time you have had vigorous, sustained inter-course for an hour? (And if it was recent, why are you bothering to read this book?) It is also true that or-gasms burn 400 calories an hour, but we repeat: If you're having hour-long orgasms four times a week, you don't have a lot to complain about and you should be sure to donate your body to science. Otherwise, according to our research, a typical orgasm uses up slightly less than 2 calories. Not even a Life Savers' worth.

5. Stretching. Feels good, doesn't use enough cal-ories to count. Don't bother unless you really like put-ting your ankle over your shoulder for its own sake.

How Many Calories You Burn While Playing Cards, Ironing a Pair of Slacks, or Engaging in Other Forms of Nontraditional Exercise

Every activity short of being dead counts as exercise as long as it is performed with gusto. Even certain forms of being dead may be metabolically beneficial if you consider that a woman who is 130 pounds burns 78 calories an hour doing nothing but *lying at ease.* Of course, a deficit of 78 calories can be wiped out in one second by eating a handful of raisins. But when was the last time you heard about a corpse having a snack? Multiply 78 calories by eternity and the number becomes significant.

The following energy expenditure chart includes a wide range of everyday household activities. (You do regard *coal mining* as an everyday pastime, don't you?) For the sake of comparison, we have also included a few sports. Unfortunately, with a few notable exceptions—*fast ax chopping* and *forking straw bales* come to mind—more calories are burned doing sports than nonsports. Still, it is nice to know that *sitting quietly* burns any calories at all, let alone a third of those burned doing *gymnastics*.

Unless specified, these numbers apply only to women. In the cases where calorie expenditures are given for both males and females, it is notable that males are more calorically taxed when it comes to carpet sweeping, cooking, knitting and sewing, skiing on soft snow, and standing quietly. Females, on the other hand, put more oomph than males do into cleaning, mopping the floor, window cleaning, and shopping. This suggests a system of labor division, but we don't want to get into that.

ACTIVITY	PERSON'S WEIGHT			
	110 LBS	130 LBS	150 LBS	190 LBS
	CALORIES BURNED PER MINUTE			
Archery	3.3	3.8	4.4	5.6
Bookbinding	1.9	2.2	2.6	3.3
Boxing, in ring	6.9	8.1	9.4	11.9
Boxing, sparring	11.1	13.1	15.1	19.1
Canoeing, leisure	2.2	2.6	3.0	3.8
Canoeing, racing	5.2	6.1	7.0	8.9
Card playing	1.3	1.5	1.7	2.2
Carpet sweeping (female)	2.3	2.7	3.1	4.1
Carpet sweeping (male)	2.4	2.8	3.3	4.5
Circuit training	9.3	10.9	12.6	15.9

	PERSON'S WEIGHT			
	110 LBS	130 LBS	150 LBS	190 LBS
ACTIVITY	CALORIES BURNED PER MINUTE			
Cleaning (female)	3.1	3.7	4.2	5.3
Cleaning (male)	2.9	3.4	3.9	5.0
Climbing hills with no load	6.1	7.1	8.2	10.4
Coal mining				
Drilling coal, rock	4.7	5.5	6.4	8.1
Erecting supports	4.4	5.2	6.0	7.6
Shoveling coal	5.4	6.4	7.3	9.3
Cooking (female)	2.3	2.7	3.1	3.9
Cooking (male)	2.4	2.8	3.3	4.1
Cycling, leisure (9.4 mph)	5.0	5.9	6.8	8.6
Dancing, ballroom	2.6	3.0	3.5	4.4
Digging trenches	7.3	8.6	9.9	12.5
Drawing (standing)	1.8	2.1	2.4	3.1
Eating (sitting)	1.2	1.4	1.6	2.0
Electrical work	2.4	3.4	3.9	5.0
Farming				
Barn cleaning	6.8	8.0	9.2	11.6
Driving harvester	2.0	2.4	2.7	3.4
Feeding cattle	4.3	5.0	5.8	7.3
Forking straw bales	6.9	8.1	9.4	11.9
Milking, by hand	2.7	3.3	3.7	4.6

	PERSON'S WEIGHT			
	110 LBS	130 LBS	150 LBS	190 LBS
ACTIVITY	CALORIES BURNED PER MINUTE			
Food shopping (female)	3.1	3.7	4.2	5.3
Food shopping (male)	2.9	3.4	3.9	5.0
Forestry				
Ax chopping, fast	14.9	17.5	20.2	25.5
Ax chopping, slow	4.3	5.0	5.8	7.3
Felling trees	6.6	7.8	9.0	11.4
Hoeing	4.6	5.4	6.2	7.8
Stacking firewood	4.4	5.2	6.0	7.6
Furriery	4.2	4.9	5.6	7.1
Gardening				
Digging	6.3	7.4	8.6	10.8
Hedging	3.9	4.5	5.9	6.6
Mowing	5.6	6.6	7.6	9.6
Raking	2.7	3.2	3.7	4.6
Golf	4.3	5.0	5.2	7.3
Gymnastics	3.3	3.9	4.5	5.7
Ironing (female)	1.7	1.9	2.2	2.8
Ironing (male)	3.2	3.8	4.4	5.5
Knitting/sewing (female)	1.1	1.3	1.5	1.9
Knitting/sewing (male)	1.2	1.4	1.6	2.0

	PERSON'S WEIGHT			
	110 LBS	130 LBS	150 LBS	190 LBS
ACTIVITY	CALORIES BURNED PER MINUTE			
Marching, rapid	7.1	8.4	9.7	12.2
Mopping floor (female)	3.1	3.7	4.2	5.3
Mopping floor (male)	2.9	3.4	3.9	4.9
Music playing				
Accordion (sitting)	1.6	1.9	2.2	2.8
Cello (sitting)	2.1	2.4	2.8	3.5
Conducting	2.0	2.3	2.7	3.4
Drums (sitting)	3.3	3.9	4.5	5.7
Flute (sitting)	1.8	2.1	2.4	3.0
Horn (sitting)	1.5	1.7	2.0	2.5
Organ (sitting)	2.7	3.1	3.6	4.6
Piano (sitting)	2.0	2.4	2.7	3.4
Trumpet (standing)	1.6	1.8	2.1	2.7
Violin (sitting)	2.3	2.7	3.1	3.9
Woodwind (sitting)	1.6	1.9	2.2	2.8
Painting, inside	1.7	2.0	2.3	2.9
Painting, outside	3.9	4.5	5.2	6.6
Plastering	3.9	4.6	5.3	6.7
Printing	1.8	2.1	2.4	3.0
Running				
11-min, 30-sec mile	6.8	8.0	9.2	11.7
9-min mile	9.7	11.4	13.1	16.6

	PERSON'S WEIGHT			
	110 LBS	130 LBS	150 LBS	190 LBS
ACTIVITY	CALORIES BURNED PER MINUTE			
7-min mile	12.2	13.9	15.6	19.1
5-min, 30 sec mile	14.5	17.1	19.7	24.9
Sitting, quietly	1.1	1.2	1.4	1.8
Skiing, hard snow				
Level, moderate speed	6.0	7.0	8.1	10.2
Skiing, soft snow				
Leisure (female)	4.9	5.8	6.7	8.4
Leisure (male)	5.6	6.5	7.5	9.5
Skindiving				
Considerable motion	13.8	16.3	18.8	23.7
Moderate motion	10.3	12.2	14.0	17.7
Snowshoeing	8.3	9.8	11.3	14.3
Standing quietly (female)	1.3	1.5	1.7	2.2
Standing quietly (male)	1.4	1.6	1.8	2.3
Steel mill, working on				
Fettling	4.5	5.3	6.7	7.7
Forging	5.0	5.9	6.8	8.6
Hand rolling	6.9	8.1	9.3	11.8
Merchant mill rolling	7.3	8.6	9.9	12.5
Removing slag	8.9	10.5	12.1	15.3
Tending furnace	6.3	7.4	8.6	10.8

	PERSON'S WEIGHT			
	110 LBS	130 LBS	150 LBS	190 LBS
ACTIVITY	CALORIES BURNED PER MINUTE			
Stock clerking	2.7	3.2	3.7	4.6
Swimming				
Backstroke	8.5	10.0	11.5	14.5
Breaststroke	8.1	9.6	11.0	13.9
Crawl, fast	7.8	9.2	10.6	13.4
Crawl, slow	6.4	7.6	8.7	11.0
Side stroke	6.1	7.2	8.3	10.5
Treading, fast	8.5	10.0	11.6	14.6
Treading, normal	3.1	3.7	4.2	5.3
Table tennis	3.4	4.0	4.6	5.8
Tailoring				
Cutting	2.1	2.4	2.8	3.5
Hand-sewing	1.6	1.9	2.2	2.8
Machine-sewing	2.3	2.7	3.1	3.9
Pressing	3.1	3.7	4.2	5.3
Tennis	5.5	6.4	7.4	9.4
Typing				
Electric	1.4	1.6	1.8	2.3
Manual	1.6	1.8	2.1	2.7
Volleyball	2.5	3.0	3.4	4.3
Wallpapering	2.4	2.8	3.3	4.1
Watch repairing	2.4	2.8	3.3	6.6
Window cleaning (female)	3.0	3.5	4.0	5.1
Window cleaning (male)	2.0	3.4	3.9	5.0
Writing (sitting)	1.5	1.7	2.0	2.5

The Skinny

Losing a Ton of Weight With Absolutely No Effort At All

Did you ever hear of the stomach flu?

TIGHT JEANS AND OTHER CLOTHES ISSUES

What motivates women to lose weight? Based on our poll, clothes are #1. (Health and men, in that order, are next.) The fantasy of fitting into that little black dress in the closet gives us the strength to say no to cheesecake. Of course, we have all been tempted to take off our tight jeans and put on those extra-large clothes that make us feel itty-bitty. We regret to inform you, however, that the waist expands to fit the elastic waistband. Big, sloppy clothes lead to big, sloppy eating. Think about it: What's another helping of mashed potatoes if you're wearing pants with wiggle-room?

But don't gigantic jeans make me look thinner? No. They make you look like you *wish* you looked thinner. They make you look baggy and saggy. They make you look like you have just dropped down to earth by parachute. They make you look like there is more of you than there is. *Are you saying that I should stuff myself into clothes made for Barbie?* No, clothes that fit too tightly look equally unflattering. And they make you feel hopelessly large, which can cause you to console yourself with food.

So what do skinny women do? They wear clothes that fit. Or they have several sets of clothes. Other clothes items:

• If you are in a consuming mood, shopping for clothes is just as satisfying as eating. Instead of lunch, try browsing through a department store. Trying on a dozen pairs of jeans in five minutes can be aerobic and just coveting the dresses you'd like to wear will make you forget about food. Plus, it's very hard to sneak pizza into the dressing room.

• According to many women, as much as 7 excess pounds can be obscured by expensive clothes.

• Make sure your clothes play up your skinniest feature and hide the others. If you are Ms. Potato Head, for example, wear a sleeveless mini-dress that shows off your lanky plastic limbs while it conceals your starchy, bulbous body.

• Venture Capitalists Take Note: We'd like to mention our skinny friend Sheila Nevins' brilliant idea—a store called Camouflage, where the clothes are arranged, not by size, but according to the body part you'd like to hide—a *Fat Ass* Department, a *Trouble in the Middle* Department, a *No Matter What I Do, I Still Have These Thighs* Department, a *Don't Look at My Stomach!* Department, an *Arms Control* Department, and so forth.

The Skinny

BEING SHORT

In case you were wondering, both of us are short and we're very bitter about it. Besides never having to shorten their pants, tall people have the clear advantage over us shorties when it comes to weight. Five extra pounds s-p-r-e-a-d over a 5'9" frame looks a lot different from five extra pounds packed—make that stuffed—onto someone 5'2".

Tall people will still whine about their misfortune ("I was so gawky when I was a kid!" "Everything's too short on me!" "I never get to wear fabulous Walter Steiger pumps!" "Men are intimidated by tall women!" "I'm always forced to see people's icky scalps!") to which we say, "Oh, *please* shut up." Short people tend toward dumpy, chunky, and stout no matter how hard they try, while tall people get to go through strapping, substantial, and she-has-a-lot-of-presence phases before anyone thinks they're fat. Their margin of weight error is much larger than a short person's. We hate them.

To cheer up our small-sized readers, remember this:

1. Tall people, even skinny tall people, wear larger sizes than skinny short people.

2. No one ever calls a tall person "petite" or "nymphlike." Ever.

3. Many, many, many men confuse shortness with thinness. This might be because most of them are taller than we are, so they have a distorted perspective from which they view women, which seems to make them see a short woman as being littler than she is. Even when you are quite fat, they get really confused and still think you're "tiny." To them, in fact, you *are* tiny—you're at least tinier than they are, circumferencewise, and your head barely reaches their armpits. That's the miracle of perspective, which is why we also love Renaissance art. Or maybe men are just stupid. Either way, it's to a short girl's advantage.

The Skinny

NAKED EATING

We have considered eating raw eggs in the hopes of picking up a touch of salmonella poisoning (an easy 14-pound loss). We have been tempted to swallow tapeworms (quite the diet rage a few years ago). We are willing to diet until we're dizzy. But Naked Eating is where even we draw the line.

Naked Eating involves eating your meals alone, in your house, in front of a mirror . . . *without clothes!* (A real pro, we suppose, might add fluorescent lights to that winning mix.) A skinny woman we know has had great success eating this way. Most days, she even manages to tear herself away from the office at lunchtime so that she can eat her tuna salad sandwich in full view of her unclad self. No doubt such a technique would discourage overeating. Probably even eating. Living, in some cases.

We hope that, thanks to this book, a Naked Eating craze will sweep the nation. We hope it spreads to dinner parties and restaurants and snack bars at airports. If so, disregard the chapter "Tight Jeans and Other Clothes Issues."

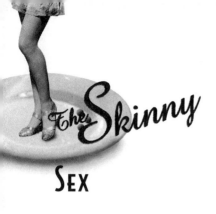

The Skinny

SEX

You may think of sex as a contact sport, but there's a reason it will never be an Olympic event. No matter how acrobatic you are in bed/in the car/in the airplane lavatory, the sexual act—from batting your eyelashes to putting your clothes back on—just doesn't burn up many calories. (Even if, one skinny woman advises, you squirm around during sex as if you were a snake and a stake had been driven through your body.) Here are the numbers:

- Kissing: 6–12 calories per kiss
- Foreplay: 100 calories per hour
- Intercourse: 100 calories per hour, if you're passive; 250 calories per hour if you're aggressive
- Orgasm: 400 calories an hour (an impressive number, but when was the last time you had an orgasm for a solid hour?)

But here's the good news. The anticipation of having sex seems to make many women eat sparingly. Also, if you're a night binge-eater, sexual congress is often exhausting (and satisfying) enough to forestall your usual refrigerator raid for at least that night. And one more thing: The caloric content of a teaspoon of semen is a mere one to five calories.

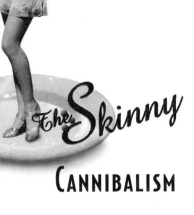

CANNIBALISM

Would you gain weight if you ate your own leg? Believe it or not, this was a topic of great interest at one Skinny Lunch. We decided—and guess what, surprisingly little scientific research has been done in this field—that you would certainly lose weight. Here's what we figured: First, we're assuming you'd eat the leg without a cream sauce and that unless you were really hungry, you'd skip the bones. Moreover a certain amount of what you ate would be, shall we say, passed through your system. And, of course, you'd be minus the leg. Not to mention the shoe. Thus, you would lose overall.

In case you were also wondering, we give the thumbs off—er, up—to the practice of eating human flesh—purely from a weight perspective, that is. Again, few studies have been done into the dietary aspects of this menu choice, but we have never seen pictures of a fat cannibal. People are just not something you want to eat too many of. Indeed, a doctor we know says that cannibals—and he claims that the only ones left these days are in Papua, New Guinea—are subsistance eaters who eat only to stay alive. In other words, they do not crave many jelly rolls. (What they do crave is calcium, which is why they boil the bones and then eat them.)

One tip when ordering: Pick the lean cuts, and, for that matter, the lean people.

The Skinny

STAMPS, MEDICINE, AND OTHER SOURCES OF HIDDEN CALORIES

If you are wary about licking a postage stamp because of the calories, rest assured that 1) there is no more than 1/10 calorie's worth of glue in a stamp and 2) the U.S. Postal Service now has self-adhesive stamps, anyway. Most of the "nutrition" in a stamp comes from carbohydrates, but even if you are on an all-protein diet, you will never get fat writing letters unless you are in the habit of eating chocolate bonbons as you compose.

Of course, we understand that counting calories is not always rational. There is, for instance, the "Gimme-a-bacon-ultimate-cheeseburger-a-sausage-croissant-fries-and-a-diet-make-sure-that-is-DIET-Coke" syndrome, whereby that measly last calorie can seem like the calorie that bloated the camel's hump. People suffering from this syndrome tend to feast until they explode, then forego the antacid because of the calories. But, let's get real. Fear of fattening medicine is not a reason to become a Christian Scientist. The only reason to become a Christian Scientist is that an untreated fever burns calories and can also kill your appetite.

Below are calorie counts for some nonfood edibles:

HYGIENE AND OVER-THE-COUNTER DRUG PRODUCTS

Crest toothpaste	12 calories per brushing (if you can't help yourself and eat up all the yummy toothpaste)
Scope	50 calories per ounce, if swallowed
Pepto-Bismol (liquid)	less than 1 calorie per adult dose
Milk of Magnesia (original or mint)	zero
Milk of Magnesia (cherry)	74 calories per 4 tablespoons
Milk of Magnesia (concentrated strawberry)	44 calories per 2 tablespoons
Advil, one tablet	less than 1 calorie
Tylenol gel caps	less than 1 calorie
Midol	zero
Vicks cough drops (cherry or menthol) in the bag	11.1 calories per drop
in the box	8 calories per drop
Flintstones One A Day Vitamins (complete formula)	3 calories
Phillips One a Day vitamins for adults	3 calories
Nyquil (liquid, cherry or original)	92 calories per ounce
IV fluid	
Saline solution	neglible

Glucose solution	varies depending on the concentration of glucose

MISCELLANEOUS

Semen	1 to 5 calories per teaspoon
Metamucil wafers (sugar-free orange)	20 calories
(apple crisp and cinnamon spice)	121 calories per dose (2 wafers)
Tums	2½ calories per tablet
Life Savers	10 calories per piece
Pez (3-oz roll)	35 calories
Sugarless Pez (3-oz roll)	30 calories
Lipstick	neglible (unless you're a lipstick-a-holic and eat the whole tube)*
Edible underwear	if you have to ask, don't eat it

*We read that over a lifetime, a woman consumes 9 pounds of lipstick. However, we could find no corroboration among cosmetics companies or dieticians.

MISERY, ANXIETY, AND DEPRESSION

God makes you miserable for a reason. It's His way of helping you slim down. So forget the adage "*No pain, no gain.*" The more pain, the more wane. Indeed, extreme emotional turmoil is the best diet we know. It kills our appetite; turns us into insomniacs who are on the treadmill every morning at five, trying to vent our anxiety; and gives us heart palpitations which are almost as good as exercising.

Unfortunately, this is not the way it always works for everyone:

1. There are people who suffer from the bad kind of depression—that is, they actually eat more when they are unhappy, hoping to find some solace in food. (See The Skinny on Prozac.) This is too sad for us to even contemplate, so we just don't.

2. And then there are some who lose under heavy-duty anxiety or depression, but gain when the stress is less severe. We asked Dr. Lorraine Eyerman, a registered dietician with a practice in Manhattan, for a physiological explanation. Mild emotional strain, she said, is linked to a serotonin deficiency. Eating certain

foods boosts our serotonin levels and thereby restores our sense of well-being. Here's the bad news: Those happy foods are carbohydrates, especially sweets, especially chocolate. Ironically, eating those happy foods makes us fat, which makes us sadder, which makes us eat more, which makes us sadder, etc., etc., etc. To stop the cycle, we advise therapy, antidepressants, or famine.

But cheer up. (Not too much, though!): If you're like most of the women we talked to, you can count on dropping some pounds if you're unhappy enough. How many? It depends on how much you're willing to suffer, but here are some guidelines, according to crisis. (Sorry, but if you are someone who gains weight when depressed, these numbers refer to pounds accrued.)

Breakup with boyfriend	6–8 pounds
Studying for the bar exams	2–4 pounds
Planning a wedding	10–12 pounds
The caterers cancel a few days before your wedding	15 pounds
Discover husband is having an affair	15 pounds
Divorce	15–18 pounds
Custody battle	16–20 pounds
Moving to a new house	10–12 pounds
About to move to a new house and the deal falls through on your old house	15–18 lbs
Your boss announces that the company is downsizing next month	13 pounds

Your sixteen-year-old son tells you he wants to drop out of school and become a professional juggler	11 pounds
Your twenty-five-year-old daughter moves back in with you	8 pounds
Death in the family	8–12 pounds
Death in the family and you inherit a million dollars	Get ready to gain a lot of weight!

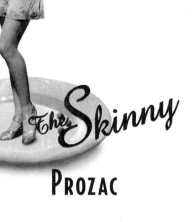

The Skinny

PROZAC

Do antidepressants make you fat or thin? In part, this depends on the type of depression you're attempting to anti. If you suffer from what is known as agitated or traditional depression, you have lucked out in the sense that you will tend to lose your appetite. Antidepressants unfortunately redress that problem and you will probably start to eat again. If, on the other hand, you have an atypical depression, you will sleep a lot, but, alas, in your moments of being awake, you will crave carbohydrates. Taking antidepressants, in this case, will make you lose weight by decreasing your appetite and increasing the amount of exercise you do. That said, there are some basic rules (and many exceptions to them because different individuals respond differently to the same drug):

- The older antidepressants—that is, the MAO inhibitors like Nardil and Parnate and tricyclides like Elavil and Tofranil—tend to cause weight gain.
- The newer antidepressants—that is, the selective serotonin re-uptake inhibitors like Prozac, Zoloft, Paxil, Luvox, and Celexa—tend to cause initial weight loss (say, 4 to 6 pounds in the first

few weeks) but after a few months your weight normalizes.

- The antidepressant Remeron makes you gain, gain, gain.
- Wellbutrin does not affect weight one way or the other.
- Lithium can make you gain weight but does not do so necessarily. Ditto for Depakote, usually prescribed for seizures and bipolar disorder and experimentally tried for chronic pain.

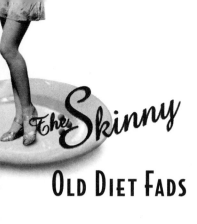

The Skinny

OLD DIET FADS

As long as there have been clothes, there have been women who wanted to wear a smaller size. And as long as there has been grapefruit and guilt, there has been a way to achieve that. Below are some of our favorite old weight-loss plans, most of them popular in the early 1900s. We swear to God we did not make these up. They seem crazy today, but who knows? What if one of them works? Even just a little.

—DIETING BY BUDGET Go ahead and eat whatever you want as long as it doesn't cost more than fifty cents a day. (This may not have been as punishing as it seems, for the diet was popular in 1889 when fifty cents was really fifty cents.)

—EATING DRY An almost no-liquid diet, that permits only one cup of black coffee at breakfast and clear tea at lunch.

—MUCOUSLESS DIET Avoid meat and flour because they produce dangerous mucus. (According to the promulgators of this plan, you know you are on the road to skinniness if you break out in boils and rashes.)

**—ROLLING AROUND ON THE FLOOR TO BRING
DOWN THE FLESH** We think the name says it all.
And by the way, not long ago, we bought a booklet in
the supermarket called *Roll Yourself Thin in Twelve
Minutes*. . . .

**—THE ONLY FIVE GALLONS OF MILK A DAY
DIET** Highly popular in 1909, an era that did not include refrigerators. Obviously, you needed to own a
cow to go on this diet.

—FLETCHERISM A method started by Horace
Fletcher, who was able to cut his food intake in half by
chewing his food so obsessively it became a tasteless
liquid. This method helps reduce food intake (and
probably the number of people willing to eat with you).

—TOBACCO Surgeon General, listen to these
words written by Clarence Lieb in *Eat, Drink, and Be
Slender* (1929): "How vastly better to smoke a cigarette while waiting for food service than to munch the
deadly bread and butter. . . . A smoke as a dessert substitute is excellent, having a satiety value equal to, if
not greater, than sweet desserts or various candies. . . .
[Smoking's] potentiality for harm is infinitesimal compared with the harm that sugar coating can do."

—HORSEBACK RIDING Once again, we quote
Clarence Lieb: "The outside of a horse is good for
both the outside and inside of a fat person . . . A lively
horse is desirable, too, because weight reduction will
be found to approximate the spirit of the animal."

—THE TAPEWORM CURE Simply swallow the
tablet containing the tapeworm and all the extra food
lying around your stomach is eaten.

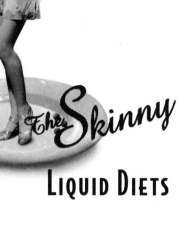

The Skinny

LIQUID DIETS

Liquid diets are the delicious, healthy way to lose weight and stay fit—well, at least that's what it says on the Slim-Fast label. As it happens, we have found this to be more or less true. The principle behind liquid diets is simple. You replace breakfast and lunch with (may we quote again?) "a delicious, healthy, nourishing diet shake" that is nutritionally balanced, low-fat, and low in calories, and you round out your day's meals with a sensible dinner.

The exact content of the diet shake depends on the brand. Most liquid diets are sold as dry mix; you add liquid and blend for your meal. Ultra Slim-Fast mix, for instance, has 120 calories and 1.5 grams of fat. After adding it to eight ounces of skim milk, it amounts to 210 calories and 1.5 grams of fat. The Dick Gregory Bahamian Diet is only 90 calories, but it is meant to be mixed with eight ounces of fruit juice, which brings it to anywhere from about 190 to 220 calories, depending on the type of juice you use. Cybergenics Quick Trim mix has 200 calories, but you can mix it with ice water, so there are no additional calories in the shake.

We know a lot of people who swear by liquid diets. They work for a couple of reasons. One is that the shakes routinize what you eat so you don't lose track of portions; if you are the sort who tends to dive into a second bowl of cereal in the morning or clean your plate at lunch, shakes are perfect for you because they leave nothing to chance or cheating. Second, they put you in that diet state of mind—you feel somehow chaste and buoyant when you're doing shakes a few times a day, which in turn makes you feel chaste and buoyant and inclined to turn down the second helping of french fries at dinner. They also put you in a soda-fountain-splurge state of mind, because being on a liquid diet means you're having chocolate milkshakes twice a day. Thirdly, there is actually some science to it. Substituting shakes for breakfast and lunch will almost certainly mean your daily calorie intake will fall (it's pretty hard to have a 220-calorie lunch made of actual food).

Also, Dr. Fried, a biochemist specializing in obesity, whom we interviewed over a high-protein, low-fat dinner one night, told us that liquid diets work in part because they disassociate you with the sensations of eating, and that seems to keep hunger in check. In other words, liquid diets get you used to the idea of not eating, so you don't think about eating as much and you don't miss it that much, either. You probably construct a food diet consisting of the same number of calories and fat contained in a liquid diet program, but apparently a food diet that is more likely to make you feel deprived and hungry, as if you were eating but just not getting as much as you want. (This is the same principle, sort of, as the idea behind single-food diets. It is a true fact that the smaller the variety of foods you eat, the less you will eat overall. Probably, we guess, because it just gets so boring.)

We've both lost weight on liquid diets, and we've both used them at times to balance out a few weeks of major indulgence. Two expense-paid weeks in Tuscany, for instance, usually spurs us to ten days of Dutch-chocolate-flavored shakes for breakfast and lunch.

What's good about them: Liquid diets are cheap, easy, reasonably tasty, are available without prescription, have lots of vitamins, are fairly satisfying, require almost no thought, aren't dangerous unless you are crazy and eat nothing but diet shakes, and will probably peel off a few pounds pretty quickly, which will get you motivated to keep losing.

What's bad: In theory, you can't do liquid diets forever (we're not sure why you can't, actually, but let's just assume you can't or shouldn't). If you aren't near a blender at lunchtime it can be a pain in the neck to figure out how to make your shake. We do see premixed canned Slim Fast in a lot of stores these days, so that's one solution; also, some of the liquid diet companies now make meal bars that can substitute for a shake, as long as you accompany it with an eight-ounce glass of milk. (Yes, you can consume fewer calories if you skip the milk, but you will then feel less full and won't be getting as much protein, etc., without the milk, and will probably start snacking sooner. Bad idea.) We've found that we lose weight only if we replace two meals with shakes rather than just one, so if you need to go out frequently for lunch, liquid diets might not be the best plan for you (we personally find a shake for dinner sort of gnarly).

Oh! Self-delusion alert! Shakes and meal bars are not anticalorie. Do not kid yourself. If you have three shakes a day plus dinner plus a couple of peanut-butter-and-chocolate-crunch diet snack bars in between you will get fat. May we quote again from the Slim-Fast Nutritional Snack Bar box?

"ATTENTION: THESE BARS ARE INCREDIBLY DELICIOUS. PLEASE DON'T OVEREAT. REMEMBER, THE PURPOSE IS TO HELP YOU KEEP YOUR WEIGHT DOWN."

Make-Your-Own Fake Shake Minus the Sweet Dairy Whey, Carrageenan, and Guar Gum

- Tablespoon or two or three of unsweetened, no-fat cocoa powder (15 calories per tablespoon)
- ¼ cup or less of nonfat powdered milk (60 calories or less)
- Artificial sweetener of your choice (oh, call it 7 calories)
- Several handfuls of ice (no guilt here)

Put everything in blender but ice. Gradually add ice until concoction is a consistency that approximates your expectations of a milkshake. Tastes kind of good.

The Skinny

Single-Food Diets

Single-food diets are the refuge of the agitated mind. In other words, if you're sick of thinking about diets, recording what you've eaten, counting micrograms, and constructing your nutritional pyramid, you may be ready for what we like to call a mono-diet. A mono-diet decrees that you eat one food product and one food product only, but you can eat as much of it as you want. There is also such a thing as modified mono-dieting, which is eat one thing and one thing only, plus a few essential extras, like lettuce, and even very modified mono-dieting, which means exclusively one food product all day, plus dinner. Mono-diets have been around since the beginning of recorded time. They are standard, in fact, in the animal kingdom. Mono-diets work because 1) the fewer different kinds of food you eat, the less you will eat in general and 2) no matter what single food you choose for your mono-diet, you will eventually get sick of it and simply won't be able to eat huge amounts of it, no matter how delicious it seemed when you started.

Popular Mono-Diets of the Past and Present:
- The Hot Dog Diet, made famous by a 1950s book of the same name. Unlimited wieners;

83

sauerkraut and ketchup provided vegetable matter; buns were optional. Big surprise: After a few hundred hot dogs, people's consumption tended to slow down. Miraculously, their weight would drop.

- The Hot-Dog-and-Beets Diet.
- The Popcorn Diet, also embraced in the fifties.
- The All-Food Diet, good for gallbladder sufferers as well as dieters.
- The Ice Cream Diet, recommended first in 1946, and today's heir apparent, the Nonfat Frozen Yogurt Diet.
- The Martini-and-Whipped-Cream Diet.
- The Non-chew Diet (not exactly a mono-diet, since you could have a variety as long as you didn't eat anything that had to be masticated, but was nevertheless monomaniacal).
- The Grapefruit Diet.
- The Frozen Grapes Diet.
- The Cantaloupe Diet.
- The Cabbage Soup Diet.

We are not saying mono-dieting is good for you— for that matter, we're not saying that anything we suggest is good for you—but it does seem to work. If you choose something sort of healthy for your mono-food—cabbage soup, say—it's probably even vaguely beneficial. On the other hand, you might as well choose something you like so that you won't feel as deprived, which is bound to happen after thirty or forty helpings of the same food. One of the skinniest women we know went on an extended homemade chocolate-chip cookie mono-diet and was very content with it. She would have salads now and then, and if she had to go out for a meal, she would order something other than chocolate-chip cookies, but otherwise she just ate chocolate-chip cookies. She lost lots of weight. Sound improbable? Consider the math. One chocolate-chip cookie has approximately 250 calories. How many could you really eat at a time? Four? Six? Or think of it this way: If that's all you were eating, you'd probably eat a few and lose interest. Maybe you'd overdo it initially, but then you're likely to level off and eat fewer and fewer, and eventually your calorie intake would be shipshape.

A better choice might be a mono-diet of something slightly less calorie-dense than cookies—nonfat yogurt perhaps, or regular yogurt, or turkey breast. But if you're going to mono-diet, you've got to surrender your logic: This is not balanced nutrition, girls, this is a peculiar, extremist diet system. Don't try to reason with it. If you are going to mono-diet, remember to: 1. Take vitamins, so that when people criticize you (which they will), you can assure them that you're taking vitamins. 2. Stick with your mono-food choice because you otherwise will gain weight (you can't, in other words, have a sausage mono-diet for breakfast, a cookie mono-diet for lunch, and a steak mono-diet for dinner; this is otherwise known as disgusting overeating and defeats the purpose). 3. Keep some goal in mind, such as "I plan to mono-diet on shrimp for a month" or "I'm having nothing but Fudgsicles for the month of August," because it will help you stick to your guns if you know it's not forever and it will help deflect those who will implore you to eat something, anything, else if you can explain that it's only for three more days or weeks or whatever.

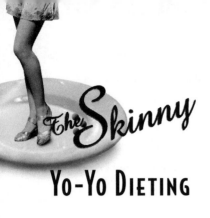

The Skinny

Yo-Yo Dieting

If someone said to you that it was a bad idea to earn a lot of money because you might lose it and have to earn it all over again, wouldn't you think they were crazy? So, if someone warns you not to lose weight because you might gain it back and have to lose it again, we suggest you apply the same judgment. All the warnings about yo-yo dieting are just crazy. First of all, none of us ever knows if the weight we lose will stay off permanently or only long enough for us to fit into that overpriced Armani evening gown, whether we lost it by the most nutritionally sound methods known to man or by using the kookiest tricks in the book. But it still doesn't mean you shouldn't try to lose weight! Secondly, science is firmly on our side: Many scientists have now determined that dieting does not permanently lower your resting metabolic rate (the energy required to keep your body alive and functioning). When you weigh less, your metabolic rate is naturally less, because you have less of a body to keep alive and functioning, but dieting doesn't permanently scramble the system. Gaining and losing weight may be frustrating, but it will not do anything hazardous other than force you to buy wardrobes in several different sizes. And thirdly, yo-yos are fun!

So why is yo-yo dieting branded as satanic? Okay, maybe some people still really think that it's bad for your body, but otherwise it's just a myth usually perpetrated by people who (just maybe) have a few pounds of their own to lose and (just maybe) feel a little guilty when you crow about your diet.

The Skinny

EATING CONSTANTLY

There are some of us who feel that a balanced diet is one in which the only balance is between the time we spend eating and the time we think about when we'll eat next; who would describe the pace of our eating as "relentless"; who believe that enough is never enough; who experience separation anxiety only when it comes to finishing a meal. You know that old saying about Chinese food—that it's great but in fifteen minutes you're hungry again? Do you feel that way about American/French/Italian/Japanese/Russian/Ethiopian/Indian/Canadian food, too?

Then you have two good options: 1) buy a straitjacket or 2) eat constantly, but cannily. The eat-every-hour-on-the-hour diet has been around since the sixties, and like a lot of other things from the sixties (bell-bottoms, Buddhism) it is ripe for revival. Here's the theory: If you love to eat constantly, you can lose weight, as long as you eat constantly but modestly. In other words, you can't eat a normal meal of 800 calories and then fifteen minutes later eat a snack of 200 calories and then fifteen minutes after that eat another 200-calorie snack and not end up looking like an ocean liner. On the other hand, if you know you're going to want to eat at regular intervals, budget your day with that in mind, and you can end up on a losing streak. First, consider the number of hours you're awake in an average day (we'll use sixteen as an example, which would account for waking up at seven and going to bed at eleven). Then figure out the number of calories you can afford if you want to lose weight (we'll say 1200). If you divide those calories up over the sixteen hours you're awake, you will see that you can eat 75 calories an hour and stay comfortably within your daily budget. Or sleep an extra hour, and you can afford 80. Or—if you're really tough—you can skip a feeding now and then, and eat 100 calories twelve times throughout the day, and you will lose weight. The only rule that you have to observe is that you can't eat normal meals—you can eat only your hourly unit. If you absolutely feel you have to eat one meallike meal in a day, you can skip a few of your allotted hourlies and bank the saved calories. (Skip the five o'clock and the six o'clock, for instance, and have a whopping 300 calories at dinnertime.) See, there's nothing wrong at all with snacking—unless you also eat normal meals. Skip the meals and you can snack like mad. And if you're going to use this plan, don't obsess about fat and carbohydrate counts. Just count to one hundred and forget about the rest.

Does a hundred calories sound measly? It's not—see the list below for hundred-calorie options. If you still think it sounds measly—well, you're on a diet, remember? Anyway, wait a mere 59 minutes and you can have another hundred-calorie extravaganza.

UNUSUAL SNACKS UNDER 100 CALORIES

5 slices of fat-free bologna
1 Dum Dum lollipop

2 T sweetened marmalade or 16 T sugar-free
  Estee or Louis Sherry marmalade

2 tsp Marshmallow Fluff

50 small radishes

2½ cups swiss chard

1 whole crab

1¼ cup salsa

4 pieces Slim Jim Big Jerk beef jerky

8–12 medium wild Eastern oysters

5 medium red peppers, without stems or seeds

1 medium mango

10 Life Savers

2 Oscar Meyer *Free* hot dogs

1 jumbo Downyflake waffle

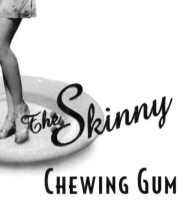

CHEWING GUM

Besides being an unsightly, irritating personal habit, chewing gum has excellent application in dieting. First of all, it is almost impossible to eat food while chewing gum unless you are some kind of wild animal. Since the first rule of dieting is Don't Eat Food, gum is therefore your friend. Some people we talked to claimed that gum made them hungry—the saliva-stimulation argument. If you are one of these people, obviously, you should not chew (and if you do, be careful about swallowing the gum because fattening food could stick to the gum in your stomach and you'd never get rid of it). For the rest of us, here are some gum topics to consider:

• One of our Skinny Lunch guests said she had lost weight on something she called The Chewing Gum Diet, which consisted of having unlimited amounts of gum for lunch, and normal meals during the rest of the day. She said gum was a good lunch substitute because it tastes pretty good, it keeps your mouth busy, and by the time you're done roaring through a package of Chiclets you might not be hungry anymore. Sounds interesting.

- We've found that nagging pangs of hunger, especially late in the day, will sometimes disappear after a few Chiclets. At least it will delay snacking, and delay (often) means you don't end up eating after all. This is very good.

- If you go to the movies with people who absolutely must eat and therefore make it hard for you to resist, chewing gum is a perfect solution. Just remember: Gum tastes terrible with buttered popcorn kernels chewed into it.

We have mixed feelings about sugarless versus sugared gum. The difference in calories is practically nothing—a stick of Care Free Sugarless, for instance, is 8 calories and 2 grams of carbohydrates; a stick of regular Beech-Nut gum is 10 calories and 2 grams of carbs. If on principle you don't eat sugar then stick with sugarless, but if you like the taste and guilty pleasure of having real gum with real sugar, you're not really doing yourself any harm by having the regular stuff. Oh, did someone say cavities? Well, they certainly don't weigh anything and while you are having the filling put in, there is no way you will be eating. Besides, Susan's dentist once told her that all gum wreaks the same havoc on your tooth enamel whether it had real or artificial sugar in it. Your own dental-health professional may have a different opinion. And who really sees your cavities, anyway?

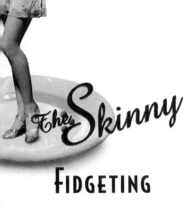

The Skinny

FIDGETING

Besides being an unsightly, irritating personal habit, fidgeting, like chewing gum, turns out to be one of the very best things an antiweight activist can do. According to Dr. Susan Fried, fidgeting really does burn calories; in fact, Dr. Fried told us that she believed fidgeting might be a key difference between thin people and fat people who appear to eat similar amounts of food. She said that a busy fidgeter might burn as many as 500 calories a day. The minute we heard this we began drumming our fingers on the table, tapping our toes, tensing and releasing our abdominal muscles, and jiggling around in our chairs. Hell of a way for an adult to behave . . . but 500 calories! That's a large nonfat frozen yogurt with a topping! And maybe topping and nuts: We later read that some people fidget away as much as 800 calories a day.

There is, of course, a chicken-and-fidgety-egg issue here. Are naturally fidgety people also naturally thin, due to some magical incendiary metabolism rather than to their dedicated fidgeting? That is, are they naturally thin anyway and they just happen to fidget? Or can constant repetitive, functionless movements actually gobble up enough calories and keep your con-

93

stitution heated up so much that you become a naturally thin person? We're going for the cheery, optimistic position that cracking your knuckles is good exercise. No matter what, there is something psychologically uplifting about fidgeting: The more you do it, the more you will think of yourself as one of those high-strung, whippet-thin neurasthenics who burns calories like a furnace. Consider the alternative. We had a private Skinny Lunch with a friend who has made dieting her avocation, and she said she thinks of herself as a very still, very stolid person who just sort of collects calories and fat in this waist-to-knee storage facility from which it never leaves. Ugh.

Better to at least picture yourself as a super-torqued engine, isn't it?

Unscientifically speaking, but based on our own fidgeting experience, the following is a suggested fidgeting program:

BEST BETS

(these use major muscle groups but are relatively inconspicuous)

- flexing and releasing thigh muscles
- alternating gluteus maximus squeezes
- pretending your waistband is on fire and you have to do everything within your power to keep your stomach from touching it

HONEST EFFORTS

(these engage less important muscles and make those around you prescribe Ritalin, but just remember: 500 calories. 500 calories. 500 calories.)

- toe-tapping
- ankle-jiggling

- knee-bouncing
- finger-drumming
- swaying side-to-side like a waterweed

Probably Useless

(but fun)
- all chewing-gum based exercise, including bubble-blowing, cracking, and pulling
- grimacing
- repeated makeup application
- taking your bracelet off and putting it back on, again and again, until you lose it
- tearing apart napkins and other paper products until the waiter gives you a dirty look
- pencil-chewing
- sniffling
- tooth-grinding

Systematic Fidgeting

(will result in a cable-knit sweater)
- knitting

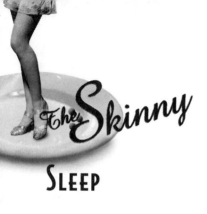

The Skinny

SLEEP

Scientists still don't know exactly why we sleep, but *we* do: It is to give the body a break from eating. Otherwise, we could gain weight twenty-four hours a day. Of course, by sleeping we don't mean eating in bed. Sleep, as we define it, is the state of not putting the Oreo that's in your kitchen into your mouth because you are dreaming of eating a more delicious Oreo. And what sweeter relief than that which comes the moment you wake up and realize you have not eaten an actual Oreo, but only a zero-calorie zero-fat figment of your imagination.

Sleep is not only the greatest appetite suppressant of all, but it actually burns calories—60 an hour. This may not be a lot of calories—you can burn up to 90 watching television!—but it is slightly more than the 50 per hour you use up driving. (We are certainly not suggesting you sleep and drive at the same time, but it's hard not to notice that the 110 calories an hour you would burn doing this is only 40 calories fewer than that used playing Ping-Pong . . . and you don't have to keep score or bend down to pick up the ball.)

Sleep is, therefore, an effortless way to lose a marginal amount of weight—marginal, that is, if you sleep normally. The women in Jacqueline Susann's *Valley of the Dolls,* in contrast, opted to be put to sleep with pills for a couple weeks so they could wake up thin. This was known as the Sleep Cure and some women actually tried it in Switzerland. In the animal kingdom, the Sleep Cure is known as hibernation. We believe that it was the real reason that Sleeping Beauty finally got the Prince. The downside of sleep, so to speak, is that you will eventually lose muscle mass, and the less muscle mass you have, the lower your basal metabolism is. Bears, after all, are not known for their slim figures.

How Can You Make Sleep Work for You?

- If you are a night binger, try to go to sleep before you start to eat. Similarly, a Skinny Luncher who tends to overeat in the afternoon, told us she takes a nap instead.
- Try to toss and turn on the theory that every iota of energy expended counts. Go to the bathroom several times a night for added exercise, but don't stop in the kitchen on the way.
- Sleep through breakfast, the refreshment portion of your airline flight, and your midnight snack. Don't sleep through your session at the gym, though.
- Some women visualize themselves thin every night as they go to sleep. This does not work for us. It makes us hungry.

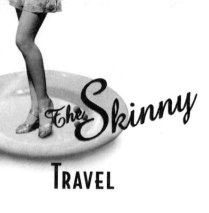

TRAVEL

Let us begin with a few travel definitions:

• "Vacationing" means going somewhere delightful and fascinating where you intend to have fun.

• "Visiting" means going somewhere that may or may not be delightful and fascinating where someone(s) you need to see happens to live. "Someone(s)" can include, but is not exclusively defined as, your parents, your in-laws, tertiary blood relations, or your spouse's college roommate.

• "Traveling" means going somewhere most likely not delightful and probably even dull because someone, usually your boss, has requested that you do so.

In order to figure out how to get or stay skinny on the road, you have to determine whether you're vacationing, visiting, or traveling, because we assure you that there are expressly different guidelines for each. However, there are a few universals:

• *Try to travel to a developing country or any country where bacteria is the national dish.* For most people, this is a guaranteed way of losing an easy eight pounds. (In fact, with this in mind, we are considering marketing bottled water from, say, India or Mexico and calling it "Montezuma's Revenge. . . .")

• *Order a low-calorie or low-fat meal when you buy your airline ticket.* They're usually terrible, but so are the regular meals, so you might as well at least feel a little virtuous right away.

• *Call ahead whenever you're staying in a hotel and ask whether the room has a minibar.* If it does, ask to be put in a room without one or to have the contents removed before you arrive. Don't be shy. If the desk clerk gives you a hard time, remember: It's just the desk clerk. Also, desk clerks have told us that people make this request all the time, so be assured that you won't be coming across as the one weirdo who demanded a room without a minibar. If you still feel shy, just say, "I have allergies and cannot have foodstuffs in my room. Please make sure there is no minibar. I can have my doctor call you if that's necessary." No one will ask for your doctor to call, by the way. Or have your travel agent make the no-minibar call; after all, that's what travel agents are for. If you arrive and there is still a minibar in your room, demand a different room immediately. Don't put your stuff down and shoo away the porter because hotels hate to move you once you've been installed in a room. Tell the porter to hang on to your bags, call down to the front desk and ask for another room. If your room has a locked minibar, do not accept the key. By the way, if you don't have any problems with eating all the food in minibars, the preceding does not apply to you.

• *Do not fear fast food.* This is not an aesthetic evaluation; it's just that sometimes, believe it or not, your best hope for a lean meal while traveling might be at a fast-food place. At the very least fast food is consistent and the restaurants usually post nutritional information (or consult The Skinny on Fast-Food Restaurants first); in the long run, a dreary broiled chicken sandwich at McDonald's is going to be a better bet than having a homestyle lard-and-potato stew pie, calorie-and-fat-content unknown, that you'll obsess over for a week.

• *If you are going somewhere with unpredictable food, throw a couple of snacks in your suitcase that can help in a pinch.* For instance, there is no such thing as a low-fat Eastern European lunch. Therefore, don't have one: Have a piece of turkey jerky or a Slim-Fast lunch bar instead and go shopping while everyone else is eating.

VACATIONING

If you're going on a vacation somewhere that has great food served in charming places—say, Paris or Siena or Marrakech—maybe dieting can wait. It's not going to kill you to eat heartily for ten days or so, no matter what: The rule of thumb is that you will lose whatever you've gained on a trip by simply returning to your normal eating habits for as many days as you spent traveling. Four-day binge in Tuscany? Four days at home eating like a civilized person will probably cancel out most of the damage. If you're going for a month, then you should worry, and you should deploy all the techniques discussed throughout the book. Less than fourteen days? Don't be a complete lunatic—i.e., don't drink straight from the olive oil bottle—but don't kill yourself if you eat a little more than you usually do. It's a vacation, for heaven's sake.

If you're somewhere that the food is good enough to be part of the vacation experience, a reasonable approach is to be judicious until dinner, and then have whatever you want. In other words, if you're going to four-star restaurants in Paris, go ahead and get something great, but just don't have four croissants for breakfast, too. Stick with a dry baguette. Or nothing. Or go to one of those super-expensive mysteriously complicated French drugstores and buy yourself a little bottle of Slim-spray, an aerosol version of appetite suppressant that we have found doesn't seem to really work but still tastes lousy, so you don't really want anything to eat after you've had your dose anyway.

If you're vacationing somewhere that has so-so food, that's a different story. Go to the Caribbean, get tan, have fun, but don't be a pig just because you're on vacation. Don't go to the breakfast buffet. Don't declare that butter is a protein substitute in the southern hemisphere. Don't order dessert at the hotel dining room: It's never any good, it's always huge, and you'll hate yourself in the morning. If you're going to have a fattening vacation, at least get fat somewhere like Italy where it's worth the pain. Overeating on hotel food in Acapulco is just stupid. If dinner is the big get-together ritual of the day, then skip breakfast altogether and try to have a low-impact lunch like a shrimp cocktail (there are shrimp cocktails at all hotels, everywhere in the universe).

Visiting

It's in-law time, or maybe it's best-college-friend visit time, or it's Passover with Great-Aunt Sadie. Yikes. If you can possibly swing it, stay in a hotel rather than being a house guest: There's less food around and fewer opportunities for people to pester you to eat. If you have to stay at someone's house, stay in bed late in order to skip breakfast—explain that you need fourteen hours of sleep (you can just stay in your room reading). Otherwise your day will begin with fourteen bagels, cream cheese, and coffee cake, and you will feel like shooting yourself. Later, suggest taking your hosts out to dinner or, better yet, suggest you'll do the cooking as a "house gift." Then whip up something lean and mean like chicken breast and green beans with nonfat frozen yogurt for dessert, or find a Yellow Pages and look up a gourmet take-out joint. Tell your hosts you love to cook. Tell them it would make you happier if you could contribute something to the household. If all else fails, pretend to be either a vegetarian or allergic to wheat throughout the visit; that'll automatically cut out a big percentage of what they'll feed you. Don't feel guilty: You're saving them money.

TRAVELING

In some ways, traveling for work is the easiest kind of skinny traveling. First of all, you're on your own. No one is going to be offended if you don't eat their Boston cream pie, and no one else is going to be annoyed if you beg off dinner at the Headcheese and Foie Gras Cafe. Business dinners can be tricky, but you can order chicken anywhere, and if everyone's drinking, no one will notice if you've left nine-tenths of your meal. If you're eating in the hotel, just remember: Just because you're lonely, bored, tired, and estranged, you don't have to order the fried seafood platter with buttered mashed potatoes. In fact, if you eat in the hotel every night, get friendly with the waiter and let him or her know you're trying to eat sparingly; they'll usually help out and even arrange for custom-ordered food if you're nice. We recommend eating in the hotel, by the way. If you venture out you're less likely to get pampered. Also, business travel usually takes you somewhere that doesn't have interesting food, and the hotel is almost always in a boring neighborhood, so why go out? Instead, use the hotel gym, get an egg-white omelet for dinner, and then go back to your room and watch pay-per-view. Refer to the first portion of the chapter for assurance that when you're in small towns or anywhere that doesn't have a highly evolved slimness consciousness, your best lunch might be a chicken salad at McDonald's. Or, stop into the local grocery store and get some cut-up vegetables or Wasa crisps or turkey breast. No, it's not fun to eat this way, but it's not as horrible as feeling like you've eaten a huge and heavy lunch when all you wanted was a little bite.

Another option is to request travel assignments only to places with lousy food—England, Scotland, Rwanda, Sudan, Antarctica. If necessary, have it written into your contract that you refuse business travel to any country with a three- or four-star restaurant.

The Skinny

SPACE TRAVEL

This is the kind of travel that is never broadening. It is, on the contrary, almost always a sure way to lose weight. In fact, while you are in orbit you are weight-LESS. Even without the help of a no-gravity environment, though, your hunger and thirst decrease, your metabolism changes, and, if you're lucky, you get motion sickness. Of course, what you lose is muscle, bone, and water, not fat. But, hey, your clothes are still baggy when you reenter earth. By the way, Tang (made by the mix) is 86 calories per 6 fluid ounces; and *really* how much can you drink?

The Skinny

MOVIES, SCARY
AND OTHERWISE

Have you ever noticed that when you watch a scary movie, your heart races, your palms sweat, your hackles stand on end, your breath becomes shallow—in other words, you have the same physiological experience that you have when you exercise? Doesn't it follow logically, then, that along with being tense and wrung out during the movie you would also burn calories, the way you do when you exercise? And doesn't it follow, then, that when you are trying to lose weight and are looking for every possible advantage, going to scary movies is worthwhile? Even if it only burns a handful of extra calories?

We think so, and we asked our diet consultant, Dr. Susan Fried, to confirm or deny. She told us that it is certainly not the most efficient way to lose weight, but that having a scary-movie terror attack probably does use some energy. Not a lot of calories, but at least one or two, and when you're counting, every single calorie counts. Another benefit: If the movie is scary enough (or sad enough or gory enough) it will probably kill your appetite for a few hours afterward, which means even more calories saved.

On the other hand, unscary movies can be treacherous. Product placement has made them just too appetizing. See Gummi Bears, eat Gummi Bears. See Gummi Bears on a high-resolution, wide screen, eat more Gummi Bears (130 calories for 18 pieces). We are convinced, too, that there are noxious subliminal messages planted in the previews that compel you to buy expensive chocolate products at the concession stand.

Speaking of noxious, it is impossible for a human being to smell popcorn and then not buy some (Aromatherapy Principle #1). No—not just *some*. Because it's such a bargain (and you should *always* avoid food bargains—see "Free Food"), you choose the largest size—the one that comes in a bucket big enough for a family of five to live inside. After all, you reason, you're sharing the popcorn so the calories don't really count. Contrary to common belief, popcorn is not devoid of calories, especially not the kind that is served in movie theaters, which, even without the additional "butter" topping, comes doused in coconut and/or palm oil (even more saturated in fat than real butter). Movie popcorn without butter is 54 to 58 calories per cup; add anywhere from 5 to 28 extra calories per cup for butter; and don't forget that the smallest size of movie popcorn is at least three cups. Moreover, popcorn has a high Calories Per Minute quotient of 52. (See The Skinny on Calories Per Minute.)

Obviously, this behavior must be stopped. How?

- If you must buy popcorn, place it on the floor by your feet so that someone will accidentally kick it over.

- Always go to the movies on a date. It is too embarrassing to overeat in front of someone you might later kiss.
- Don't ever buy the loose candy. It is a scientific fact that you will fill the bag with candy till the point right before it bursts.
- The best kind of candy to buy are JuJubes. You will automatically throw out the greens and the purples. Moreover, each piece has a mere $2^3/_4$ calories, and because they inevitably get stuck in your teeth, you cannot eat too many.
- Take no money to the theater (buy your ticket with a credit card) and do not go out for a bite afterward.
- Don't ever go to the movies when you're hungry.
- Never go to a movie that features food. Until Congress publishes a PG-Fattening movie rating system, we offer you these specific movies to avoid: *Babette's Feast, Eat Drink Man Woman, Big Night, Tom Jones, Fried Green Tomatoes, Bread and Chocolate, Kentucky Fried Movie,* and all Italian movies.
- If you have to see a hunger-inducing movie, at least try to wait until you have stomach flu or a hangover or a first-trimester pregnancy.
- Failing that, make it a double-feature, and make sure the second one is an homage to *Nightmare on Elm Street.*

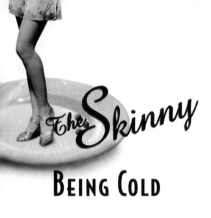

The Skinny

BEING COLD

If scary movies burn up a few calories, not many but a few, what about shivering? Our sources informed us that there is a practice among seriously diet-conscious girls to venture outside in the dead of winter wearing the skimpiest of clothes, on the theory that shivering makes you lose weight. As for the validity of that reasoning, here's what we discovered: Shivering is no doubt marginally aerobic, but so is fanning yourself in the heat, or turning on the air conditioner, for that matter. Exposure to cold weather does seem to make your body work harder to maintain heat, which raises your metabolism . . . but only a smidge. So throw away the Siberia travel brochures and put on some clothes.

Now, what about the claim that ice water burns calories? We could find no doctor to support this (though we did discover that hot water weighs more than cold). Alas.

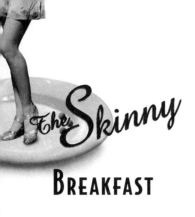

The Skinny

BREAKFAST

You know how most diets begin with that great old diet proverb: Thou Shalt Never, Ever Skip Breakfast? Well, it's nonsense. There is nothing magical about breakfast. All the preaching about blood sugar and insulin spikes and neurochemistry and metabolism is nonsense, too. If you wake up hungry, eat something. If you wake up not hungry, don't eat. Simple!

Even a clinical nutritionist at Mt. Sinai Hospital—they're the ones who always warn you against missing breakfast—was quoted recently saying that you can delay eating until you're hungry with no ill consequences. Then she added what we've suspected all along: Some people find that eating in the morning triggers their appetites and leads them to overeat throughout the day.

If you skip breakfast, just remember to eat at some point in the day before you are so ravenous that you eat something stupid. Otherwise, take pride in the fact that by skipping breakfast you are 1) saving a bunch of calories, 2) saving time, 3) getting to sleep in for at least an extra eighteen minutes, and 4) maintaining your toothpaste-fresh breath for much longer than anyone who eats breakfast.

By the way, many people who are used to eating

breakfast think they will simply faint from hunger if they go without. Many of these people have never even tried to skip breakfast. Chances are, if you have any weight to lose, you will not suddenly collapse from malnutrition if you wake up, have a cup of coffee, and not eat anything until lunch. If you really are one of those people who wakes up starving, do what you need to do, but if you eat breakfast out of habit, try avoiding it for a few days and see what happens. Or don't eat right when you wake up—wait until mid-morning, when you'll probably eat less than you would first thing because you're busier. If you still insist on eating breakfast, at least be careful. A lot of typical breakfasts look innocuous but aren't. Perfect example: cereal.

Eaten in the precious, precise quantities listed as "serving size," many cereals are fat-free and have about 110 calories. However, eaten in the quantities a normal person eats, you're getting no bargain. Three-quarters of a cup of cornflakes? Who do they think they're kidding? A regular bowlful is closer to two cups, and even then you secretly want more.

Actually, all high-carbohydrate breakfasts are Chinese-food-like in their tendency to never quite satisfy you and then make you hungry again in fifteen minutes. Therefore, breakfasts of pancakes, cereal, waffles, sweet rolls, donuts, muffins, toast, or bagels are a bad idea. The one exception to this is oatmeal, which is digested more slowly than ordinary carbs, so you don't get hungry again as quickly. Also, who can really overeat oatmeal?

Protein at breakfast? Definitely, as long as it's not too fatty. Egg whites scrambled or made into an omelet; nonfat cottage cheese (sprinkle with sweetener and cinnamon and you'll think you're eating some-thing really good); or nonfat yogurt are good break-fasts. And before you shriek in horror, consider having something that's not typically breakfast-y, like turkey or chicken or fish. It's not that different from having sausage or bacon or a ham omelet—which you shouldn't have, of course, because they're pure fat, but they do prove that a savory rather than sweet breakfast is not a sin against nature. Remember—Japanese people eat soup and fish for breakfast every day and they're skinny.

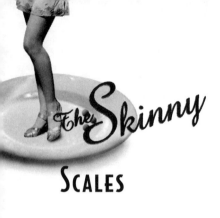

The Skinny

SCALES

Nothing, with the possible exception of the existence of God, has been debated as strenuously and ardently as the issue of weighing yourself while dieting. We polled our participants at the Skinny Lunches and found an almost consistent 50/50 split—that is, some people weighed themselves about fifty times a day, and everyone else never weighed themselves and planned to stay off a scale for at least fifty more years.

The fact is, there is no middle ground. Most credible diet advisers will tell you to weigh yourself in moderation—once a week or every other day—but we completely disagree. Weight fluctuates constantly. If you get on a scale occasionally, like a normal person would, you aren't getting an average number; you're getting a random number that reflects what you just ate, how much water you just drank, whether or not you've just had your period, how recently you've gone to the bathroom, the time of day, the force of gravity on the earth's superheated inner core, etc. If you hit it at a bad moment, you'll be more depressed than you maybe need to be. If you get lucky and weigh in at an unusually low point, you will be filled with a false and dangerous sense of satisfaction.

Which means what? Which means that you should

go to one extreme or another: Weigh yourself constantly or never. If you decide on constantly, make it a fetish. Weigh yourself when you first wake up but after you've peed; weigh yourself before and after exercise, weigh yourself after dinner, before bed. It's fun. In a day your weight can bounce around several pounds. Over a week or so, you will probably see some kind of overall pattern of generally up or generally down and you can base your mood on that. True, when you have an unusual spike up or down you're going to have a fit, even if you know that when you weigh yourself again in a few hours, the trend might reverse, but after a few months of hopping on and off the Terraillon, you'll develop a kind of scale wisdom.

One of our Lunchers said she weighed herself three times a day on three different scales—one at home, one at the gym, and one at work (at work? this girl's serious). We salute her, but only if she can keep the three scales separate in her mind, since we know and you know that individual scales do vary. Another Luncher said she traveled with her own scale, so she could avoid stepping on an unfamiliar or unreliable one. (Travel tip: Send scales through as luggage, not carry-ons. They're heavy.) And another Weigher said she always kept a scale in the front seat of her car so she could hop out and weigh herself whenever the urge struck. She noticed that she lost the most weight after a long day doing the outlet stores. Still another Weigher told us that she gets up at six A.M., weighs herself, and if she's not happy about the number, she goes back to bed for an hour and a half and weighs herself again. She swears she can "lose" up to two pounds that way. (For the anal-compulsive Weighers: According to a couple doctors we consulted, you can deduct 1 to 3 pounds from your weight if you are constipated.)

If you are going to weigh yourself, we advise a good scale. The digital ones seem to be the best. Talking scales are an abomination and should be avoided; scales that show you what you weighed the last time you got on seem unnecessarily reproachful and gimmicky. There are ways to trick a scale—hop on and off really fast, lean against a wall, stand on one leg, hire a child to stand in for you—but remember, dear Weighers, you're only cheating yourself.

Now, for the opposition view. NEVER, EVER, UNDER ANY CIRCUMSTANCE, WEIGH YOURSELF. As it happens, both of us are former incessant Weighers who've undergone conversion experiences and now forswear scales altogether. Why? Because 1) weighing yourself constantly takes up too much time and can begin to interfere with other activities such as work, domestic responsibilities, television viewing, and eating; and 2) what you weigh and how fat you actually feel often don't correspond, and you have to choose which of these you plan to pay attention to, because you really can't do both. In other words, you have to live by scale numbers or live by the fit of your jeans, and we finally decided the fit of our jeans was fundamentally more meaningful, except to an insurance actuary. And who cares about insurance actuaries?

If a doctor insists on having you get on a scale, either refuse (let his HMO sue you) or stand backward and tell the smirking nurse that you don't want her to say anything, especially anything like "Wow, at this rate, you'll weigh 200 before the end of the year!" If you have to fill in forms that request your height and weight, just make up a number. It doesn't matter what you say, really. The only time it might matter is when you're about to be anesthetized and you want to be sure you get the right dose. Lowballing your weight might mean you'll wake up in the middle of your heart/lung transplant; overestimating your weight might mean you'll wake up never. You might want to have the anesthesiologist weigh you—just stand backward and tell him or her not to announce the results. By the way, if you feel foolish telling your doctor you don't want to be weighed or don't want to be told the number, get over it. Doctors hear this all the time. One more thing: If you're planning to fly on a small, single-engine plane where exact passenger load matters, maybe you should consider taking a train.

Being a nonscaler doesn't mean quitting all forms of measurement. Everyone we talked to who doesn't weigh herself has some other way of tracking her weight, the most popular one being the fit of a particular pair of pants. If you have even the slightest amount of personal integrity, you can put on a pair of pants and tell exactly how tight or loose they feel. You can also keep track of your weight by checking the way your rings fit, although water retention affects your fingers acutely—you can be losing weight but have your rings feel tight if you've had a lot of salt in the last day or two. (Also, what if you're losing weight in your fingers only? At least pants tend to take into account parts of your body you actually care about.) Shoes, clothes with any more than .05 percent Lycra, underwear, and sweat suits are not good surrogate scales. If you choose to use jeans, you must decide in advance whether to keep one pristine pair that you never wear and never wash and therefore can trust as unchangeable. If you're going to measure yourself with a pair that you actually wear, remember that jeans shrink when they're first washed and stretch after they've been worn. It doesn't matter which of these conditions your test pair is in as long as you're consistent. And we mean really consistent: Jeans worn for two weeks straight will be a lot more stretched out than jeans worn once or twice. If you're really exacting, you can also skip the pants and measure your thighs or calves, although if you're going to do that, you might as well get on a scale. By the way, clothes do not shrink on their own. Also, if your pants suddenly seem to be getting short, you, sadly, are not getting taller: You are getting a bigger waist, butt, and thighs, and the material is hitching up.

The Skinny

EATING OUT

There are two approaches to eating at restaurants: One involves maximum intake ("Hey, honey, the bread is free!"); the other, minimum intake ("Waiter, there's a calorie in my soup"). While we don't expect you to practice total abstinence at an establishment of food, we do advise leaning toward the latter approach. Here's how:

- *Never eat beforehand.* Some people do, believing that it will make them less ravenous at the restaurant. In our experience, though, arriving at a table with a little food in our stomachs only gives us eating momentum and makes us want to fill our stomachs much sooner than we would if we had come hungry.
- *Don't order both an appetizer and a main course unless you are on a first date with a man you hope to see on a second date.* Men like women to eat but never gain weight. In other words, men like the illusion of hearty eating. This can be accomplished by ordering everything on the menu but touching only a fraction of what is on your plate. (Believe us, people notice only what you order, not what you eat.)

- *If you really don't want to eat, say that you just came from the dentist.*
- *Don't use the excuse that you just ate.* This makes you seem like you are rude, idiotic, or a liar.
- *The more expensive the restaurant, the smaller the portions.* Avoid any restaurant that features an all-you-can-eat item.
- *If you want to try a new restaurant, go with girlfriends who are on a diet.* Under such circumstances, you will feel too embarrassed to order high-calorie dishes, and perfectly within your rights to ask the waiter to substitute steamed spinach for the cottage fries.
- *Don't be afraid to give the waiter detailed instructions about how you want your food prepared.* If you'd like sauce on the side, say so even at the risk of causing your waiter to turn up his nose. A woman at one of our Skinny Lunches brought her own fat-free nonstick cooking spray and asked that the chef use that instead of butter when making her omelette.
- *No matter what you have told the waiter and no matter what the waiter told you, assume there is butter on everything—even the silverware.*
- *Never eat from other people's plates, but welcome others eating from yours.*
- *Never take home a doggie bag unless you are a doggie.*
- *When all else fails, order roast chicken.* Take the skin off and skip the mashed potatoes.
- *And, of course, never touch the bread.*

The Skinny

FAST-FOOD RESTAURANTS

Wouldn't you really rather have a hard-boiled egg, a glass of spring water, and, for dessert, a multivitamin than a couple orders of fries and a shake? If you answered yes, then you have no need for this book. But if you, like one woman we talked to, crave Whoppers so much that you once phoned the mayor of your city (Rudolph Giuliani and New York, respectively), demanding he zone more Burger Kings into your neighborhood, then you should read the following good news.

Fast food can clog your arteries and rot your teeth. Whoops. We were going to give you the good news weren't we? The good news is that if you make informed choices when ordering, you can eat at a fast-food restaurant and not walk out looking like a walking ham. That's not all the good news. Because fast-food restaurant chains operate the way tractor factories did under the centralized economy of the USSR, the Extra Tasty Crispy drumstick at the Kentucky Fried Chicken in Des Moines is the same Extra Tasty Crispy drumstick at the Kentucky Fried Chicken in Paris, in terms of size, nutritional values, and grease. Plus, all essential information—serving size, calories, calories from fat, total fat, saturated fat, sodium, protein, and carbohydrates—is publicized somewhere in the restaurant (look for a cheese- and chocolate-stained piece of paper below the How to Perform the Heimlich maneuver poster).

The real danger of fast-food restaurants is that they are fast. (For the danger of velocity in eating, see The Skinny on Speed [2] and The Skinny on Calories Per Minute.) Only a few seconds after you order, you can hold in your hands enough food to ruin forever your chances of wearing a pair of shorts in public again. If you're fleet, you'll have gobbled it down before your server has tallied it up at the cash register. In expensive sit-down restaurants, on the other hand, you basically waste the night away before they bring your meal. It is a good idea, therefore, to pick the longest line and if you're lucky, you will become so impatient, you will leave before it is your turn.

Or you can heed the following rules. Skip the sauces. Peel off the skin. Forget anything breaded or fried. Avoid sizes with the following words in them: deluxe, jumbo, colossal, king, biggie, and big-as-the-steadily-expanding-universe. Don't buy more than one of anything. Nothing with the word "blue" or "bleu" or bacon. Indulge in the low-calorie, free condiments—pickles, mustard, ketchup, pepper, napkins. Never eat as much as you can hold in your hands.

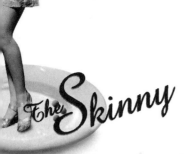

THE BEST AND WORST CHOICES IN FAST FOOD

ARBY'S (WHERE BEEF STOCK AU JUS IS ONLY 5 CALORIES AN OUNCE)

<u>Skinny Pickings (under 200 calories)</u>

- Side Salad (3 oz)—23 calories
- Lumberjack Mixed Vegetable Soup (8 oz)— 90 calories
- Roast Chicken Salad (14.4 oz)—149 calories
- Chocolate Chip Cookie (1 oz)—125 calories

<u>Chubby Choice</u>

- Philly Beef 'n Swiss Sandwich (10.4 oz)— 755 calories
- Deluxe Baked Potato (15.3 oz)—726 cal
- Triple Cheese Melt Sandwich (8.4 oz)—720 calories
- Blue Cheese Salad Dressing (2 oz)—290 calories

BLIMPIE (THE NAME SAYS IT ALL)

<u>Skinny Pickings</u>

- Salsa (.75 oz)—5 calories
- Grilled Chicken Salad (without dressing) (16.3 oz)—350 calories (so just eat half)

<u>Chubby Choice</u>

- Ham, Salami, Provolone Sub, 6 in.—590 calories

- Tuna Sub, 6 in.—570 calories
- Steak and Cheese Sub, 6 in.—550 calories

BOSTON MARKET
Skinny Pickings
- Chicken Gravy (1 oz)—15 calories
- Steamed Vegetables (²/₃ cup)—35 calories
- Fruit Salad (³/₄ cup)—70 calories
- Chicken, white meat (no skin or wing), ¼ chicken, 3.7 oz—160 calories

Chubby Choice
- Ham and Turkey Club Sandwich, with cheese and sauce (13.5 oz)—890 calories
- Meat Loaf Sandwich, with cheese (13.5 oz)—860 calories
- Original Chicken Pot Pie (1 pie, 15 oz)—750 calories
- Stuffing (¼ cup)—310 calories

BURGER KING
Skinny Pickings
- Pickles (.5 oz)—0 calories
- Side Salad (4.7 oz)—60 calories
- Broiled Chicken Salad (10.6 oz)—200 calories

Chubby Choice
- Double Whopper with Cheese Sandwich (13.1 oz)—960 calories
- BK Big Fish Sandwich (8.9 oz)—700 calories
- Strawberry Shake, medium (12 oz)—420 calories
- Mayonnaise (1 oz)—210 calories

DAIRY QUEEN (BEWARE OF ANYTHING SIZED "REGULAR" HERE)
Skinny Pickings
- Dairy Queen Fudge Bar (2.3 oz)—50 calories

- Dairy Queen Vanilla Orange Bar (2.3 oz)—
  60 calories
- Dairy Queen Lemon Freez'r ($1/2$ cup, 3.25 oz)—
  80 calories
- Hot Dog (3.5 oz)—240 calories (okay, so it's
  over 200; but it tastes so good . . .)

Chubby Choice

- Chocolate Chip Cookie Dough Blizzard, regular
  (16 oz)—950 calories
- Chocolate Malt, regular (20 oz)—880 calories
- Chicken Strip Basket with Gravy (13 oz)—860
  calories
- DQ Homestyle Ultimate Burger (9.5 oz)—
  670 calories

DOMINO'S (HOLD THE PIZZA)

Skinny Pickings

- Canned mushroom topping for pizza—2 calories
- Onion topping for pizza—3 calories
- Green pepper topping for pizza—3 calories
- Garden Salad, small—22 calories

Chubby Choice

- Marzetti Ranch Salad Dressing (1.5 oz)—
  266 calories
- Any pizza, for instance:
  —Deep Dish Medium 12" Pizza (2 slices,
    6.2 oz)—467 calories
  —Hand Tossed Medium 12" Pizza (2 slices,
    4.9 oz)—349 calories
  —Thin Crust Medium Pizza ($1/4$ pizza, 3.7 oz)—
    273 calories

HARDEE'S

Skinny Pickings

- Gravy (1.5 oz)—20 calories

- Mashed Potatoes (4 oz)—70 calories
- Grilled Chicken Salad (11.5 oz)—150 calories
- Vanilla Cone (4 oz)—170 calories

Chubby Choice

- Big Country Breakfast with Sausage (11.5 oz)—1000 calories
- Frisco Burger (8 oz)—720 calories
- Cravin Bacon Cheeseburger (8 oz)—690 calories
- Sausage and Egg Biscuit (12 oz)—630 calories

JACK-IN-THE-BOX (THERE'S A REASON JACK IS IN THE BOX: HE'S TOO FAT TO COME OUT!)

Skinny Pickings

- Soy Sauce (.3 oz)—5 calories
- Ketchup (.3 oz)—10 calories
- Grape Jelly (.5 oz)—40 calories
- Taco (2.8 oz)—190 calories

Chubby Choice

- Bacon Ultimate Cheeseburger (10.5 oz)—1150 calories
- Bacon and Cheddar Potato Wedges (9.4 oz)—800 calories
- Egg Rolls, 5-piece (10 oz)—730 calories
- Sausage Croissant (6.4 oz)—670 calories

KENTUCKY FRIED CHICKEN (NOT AS BAD AS YOU'D THINK)

Skinny Pickings

- Green Beans (4.7 oz)—45 calories
- Mean Greens (5.4 oz)—70 calories
- Tender Roast Chicken Breast, without skin (4.2 oz)—169 calories

Chubby Choice

- Chunky Chicken Pot Pie (13 oz)—770 calories
- Hot and Spicy Chicken Breast (5.9)—530 calories

Little Caesar's (AND YOU SHOULD SEE BIG CAESAR!)

Skinny Pickings

- Tossed Salad (8.5 oz)—116 calories
- Antipasto Salad (8.4 oz)—176 calories
- Cheese Pizza (1 slice)—181 calories

Chubby Choice

- Meatsa Sandwich (15 oz)—1036 calories
- Pepperoni Sandwich (1.2 oz)—899 calories

McDonald's

Skinny Pickings

- Garden Salad (6.2 oz)—35 calories
- Grilled Chicken Deluxe Salad (7.5 oz)—120 calories
- Hash Browns (1.9 oz)—130 calories
- English Muffin (1.9 oz)—140 calories

Chubby Choice

- Arch Deluxe with Bacon (8.7 oz)—590 calories
- Big Mac (7.6 oz)—560 calories
- Filet Fish Deluxe (8 oz)—560 calories
- French Fries, Super Size (6.2 oz)—540 calories

Pizza Hut

Skinny Pickings

- Thin 'N Crispy Ham Pizza (1 slice)—184 calories
- Thin 'N Crispy Veggie Pizza (1 slice)—186 calories
- Cheese Bigfoot Pizza, medium (1 slice, 2.7 oz)—186 calories

Chubby Choice

- Meat Lover's Pan Pizza (1 slice)—340 calories
- Pepperoni Personal Pan Pizza (9 oz)—637 calories
- Supreme Personal Pan Pizza (11.5 oz)—722 calories

SUBWAY

Skinny Pickings

- Veggie Delight Salad—51 calories
- Turkey Breast Salad—102 calories
- Ham Salad—116 calories
- Roast Beef Salad—117 calories

Chubby Choice

- Tuna Sub, 6 in.—542 calories
- Pizza Sub—464 calories
- Classic Italian, 6 in. BMT—460 calories

TACO BELL

Skinny Pickings

- Green Sauce (1 oz)—5 calories
- Cinnamon Twist (1 oz)—140 calories
- Taco (2.75 oz)—170 calories
- Light Chicken Soft Taco (4.25 oz)—180 calories

Chubby Choice

- Taco Salad with Salsa (19 oz)—840 calories
- Nachos BellGrande (10.75 oz)—740 calories
- Mexican Pizza (7.75 oz)—570 calories
- Bacon Cheeseburger Burrito (8.25 oz)—
  560 calories
- Seven-Layer Burrito (10 oz)—540 calories

WENDY'S

Skinny Pickings

- Hamburger Patty (2 oz)—100 calories
- Grilled Chicken Fillet (3 oz)—110 calories
- Deluxe Garden Salad (10 oz)—110 calories
- Chili, small (8 oz)—210 calories (spill 10
  calories' worth before eating)

Chubby Choice

- Taco Salad (7.4 oz)—590 calories

- Frosty Dairy Dessert, large (20 oz)—570 calories
- Big Bacon Classic Sandwich (10 oz)—570 calories
- French Fries, Biggie (5.6 oz)—460 calories

Best and Worst of Fast Food, Individual Items

- Plain Hamburger, fewest calories—McDonald's: 260 calories
- Plain Hamburger, most calories—Roy Rogers: 343 calories
- Plain Hamburger, fewest calories per ounce— Dairy Queen (59 calories per ounce)
- Plain Hamburger, most calories per ounce— Jack-in-the-Box and Roy Rogers (each 77 calories per ounce)
- Worst Way to Start the Day—Hardee's Big Country Breakfast with Sausage: 1000 calories
- Best Way to Start the Day, not including coffee—2 pieces of bacon from Carl's Jr.: 40 calories
- Dessert, fewest calories (not counting fruit)— Dairy Queen Fudge Bar (2.3 oz): 50 calories
- Dessert, most calories—Dairy Queen Chocolate Chip Cookie Dough Blizzard, regular (16 oz): 950 calories
- Shake, fewest calories—Burger King Chocolate Shake: 320 calories
- Shake, most calories—Dairy Queen Chocolate Shake, regular: 770 calories
- Shake, fewest calories per ounce—Carl's Jr. Vanilla Shake: 24.2 calories (McDonald's 2nd fewest: 29 calories)
- Shake, most calories per ounce—Dairy Queen Chocolate Shake: 85 calories

- Cheese Pizza Slice, fewest calories—Domino's Deep Dish Large Tossed Pizza: 159½ calories (2.4 oz)*
- Cheese Pizza Slice, most calories—Supreme Pan Pizza: 311 calories
- French Fries, least calories per order—McDonald's, small: 210 calories
- French Fries, most calories per order—Jack-in-the-Box Super Scoop: 610 calories
- French Fries, least calories per ounce—Hardee's: 70 calories
- French Fries, most calories per ounce—Arby's: 98 calories
- Most Fattening Pizza Topping at Domino's—Bacon: 75 calories
- Two Most Caloric Ice Cream Flavors at Baskin-Robbins—Peanut Butter 'n Chocolate, Reese's: each 180 calories per ½ cup.
- Least Caloric Ice-Cream Flavor at Baskin-Robbins—Strawberry Very Berry: 120 calories per ½ cup
- Least Caloric Light Ice Cream at Baskin-Robbins—Double Raspberry: 90 calories per ½ cup
- Least Caloric Ice Cream with No Sugar at Baskin-Robbins—Berries and Banana: 80 calories per ½ cup
- Least Caloric Reduced Sugar No-Fat Frozen Yogurt at Baskin-Robbins—all have 80 calories except Triple Delight Berry, which has 90 calories

By the way, adding cheese and mayo to a burger almost triples the calories

*Misleading as Domino's is the only pizza place that lists ounces and the forementioned is probably smaller than other pizza slices.

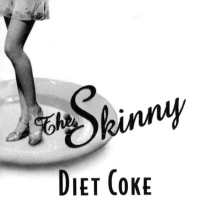

The Skinny

Diet Coke

Try as we might, we can't think of a single thing wrong with diet Coke. It has no calories, no fat, no carbohydrates, no protein—it's a perfectly balanced nonfood! Vitamin DC, as we like to call it, has gotten many a dieter through tough times. It sort of fills you up, it has that lively caffeine afterburn, it tastes like something you want to eat rather than something you *have* to eat, and—perhaps Vitamin DC's most important contribution to the dieting cosmos—it keeps your mouth busy with something other than Snickers bars.

Will a Steady Consumption of Diet Coke Overexpose You to Aspartame?

Perhaps, but if that worries you, you aren't really serious about losing weight. Until you can say with aplomb "I believe aspartame is a health food," you aren't serious about losing weight. Call us when you're really ready.

Can Too Much Diet Coke Give You a Harmful Caffeine/Red Blood Cell Ratio?

First of all, define "harmful." Secondly, use your own judgment. If you've gnawed off the corners of your desk in a fit of nervous energy, you might want to cut back a couple of six-packs.

P.S. We thought of something wrong. A liter of diet Coke, when spilled directly on the keyboard of your laptop computer will cause severe damage. Then again, you will lose weight due to the anxiety.

The Skinny

What to Do if You Accidentally Drink a Coke Instead of a Diet Coke

Consult your physician immediately.

No, Really. What to Do if You Accidentally Drink a Coke Instead of a Diet Coke

First of all, calm down. Chances are you took only a single sip before realizing your grave mistake. This is approximately five calories, the equivalent of half a Life Saver. But let's assume the worst: you were ravenously thirsty, you took a swig, you thought, "Why, I have never tasted a cola quite as delicious as this one—so crisp, so sublimely carbonated, so witty, surely a vintage year!" Then you tossed back the entire can, all 12 corn-syrupy ounces. Instead of consuming approximately zero calories (diet Coke), you squandered 97 calories (Classic Coke). You could have eaten a 3 Musketeers bar, 1/24 of a Betty Crocker Golden Pound Cake, a cup of caramel popcorn, an ear of corn on the cob, 49 small radishes, a sausage serving, or 9 7/10 Life Savers.

That isn't the point, though. It's the principle. You are 97 unwanted calories down (or is it up?) for the day, calories you had no intention of wasting at that time in that way. The devil force fed you those calories. And now you have a few options. You could throw up your hands, decide that as long as you have ingested 97 calories, you may as well ingest 9700 calories, and then devour all the food in your house. We have done that. Alternatively, you could blame whomever served you the evil potion, even threatening to sue. For added effect, tell your waitress/host/stewardess/spouse/date that you are diabetic. We've done that too.

Of course, you could also be reasonable, a route we have yet to explore. You could remind yourself that 97 calories extra in a single day does not do very much damage as long as you STOP RIGHT NOW. Moreover, as Dr. Susan Fried told us, it is more meaningful to look at the calories you consume over the course of a week than in twenty-four hours. Just as your checkbook does not revert to zero every morning, so your body does not start over simply because you go to sleep at night. Seen as part of a week-long total, 97 calories is peanuts . . . well, maybe not peanuts . . . celery sticks.

By the way, no matter how wretched you feel about the 97 calories, try not to let others know. Your handsome blind date, for one, will not be sympathetic when you tell him that due to the droplets of real Coke which have just sullied your body, your life is ruined beyond repair.

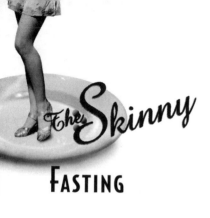

The Skinny

FASTING

Crackpots, as a rule, have a lot to say about fasting. They claim it can cure migraines, asthma, multiple sclerosis, peptic ulcers, arthritis, hay fever, the common cold, gonorrhea, prostate enlargement, impotence, deafness, as well as prevent insect bites. One book we read even prescribed fasting as a means of putting *ON* pounds for those who are dangerously underweight and unable to assimilate food (ahh, our hearts go out . . . not at all). Advocates of fasting cite references in the Bible, the Koran, the sacred texts of Buddhism and Hinduism, and probably also episodes of *Star Trek* to support their lifestyle. Talk to a New Ager and he will tell you that fasting cleanses your body, mind, and spirit. If you could ask Mrs. Gloria Lee Byrd, author of two books on outer space, why she fasted she would explain that she had been ordered by J.W., a sovereign from Jupiter, to go without food in order to bring about peace. But you can't ask her. She died sixty days into her mission.

As you might have guessed, we're more interested in losing a few pounds than world peace or even personal calm. And barring extreme surgical procedures, fasting is the most rapid method toward that end we know. It is generally estimated that a person of average weight can lose between 2 to 3 pounds per day during the early stages of a fast; and a heavier person can lose even more. Of course, as fasting detractors point out, much of this weight is water weight. That's okay; we'll take it. Did you ever hear anyone say, "Oh, she may look thin all right, but she's not actually thin—she's just missing some water"? And as for the argument that the weight will come back after the fast is over, that's fine with us, too. We would rather be skinny for a short while than not skinny at all. Besides, being skinny for a few days inspires us to make it last and/or really—this time, we mean it—eat healthily from then on.

With this in mind, we visited a spa specializing in supervised juice fasts. We asked one of the nutritionists how long we should refrain from solid food. "Everyone's juicing experience is different," she said. "It depends on why you are juicing." We stated our purpose. "Oh, no! We don't recommend juicing for weight loss," the nutritionist said, a bit miffed by our vanity. "The intent of juicing is detoxification. Juicing will help you get in touch with a meditative state of mind." While you are juicing, the theory goes, your body is relieved of its digestive responsibilities and can therefore concentrate on purging you of all the horrible impurities—physical and otherwise—lurking inside. (Say the word "juicing" enough and it will start to sound disturbingly obscene.)

We decided to juice for three days because that was how long we could survive without phones and television, neither of which were provided in our rooms. For the next nine meals, our waitperson served us a variety of juices—16 ounces per meal—at the specially reserved Juicing Table. We tried green vegetable (100 calories), carrot beet (205 calories), carrot apple beet (240 calories), watermelon (240 calories), and mixed fruit (240 calories). The cantaloupe juice (240) was best; the tomato vegetable (85 calories) was most like water. We were allowed to supplement our juice rations with limitless quantities of potassium broth, but were never tempted to do so.

During our stay at the spa, there was only one other woman juicing. She was juicing for eight days because, she told us, it made her feel wonderful. On the morning of our second day and her sixth day, we observed her hand trembling as she squeezed a lemon into her hot water. That day at lunch, as we gulped down our apple lemon ginger and parsley juice (240 calories) and she nursed her grapefruit juice, mixing it with water to make it last longer, she reprimanded us for standing as we drank, explaining that juicing works much better if you sit. She was similarly upset when she learned we were not having the colonics because, according to her, that, too, is crucial to the juicing experience. We thought it best not to let her know that we had driven to town our first night to buy a three-day supply of diet Coke.

How much did we lose? One of us lost five pounds, the other six. (We're too competitive to tell you who lost more.) We never felt lethargic. We never even felt hungry after the first twelve hours or so. However, our carpal tunnel syndrome did not disappear; nor did our athlete's foot. J.W. from Jupiter never talked to us about peace in the universe, though we would have welcomed the diversion. Fasting is boring; who would have guessed that chewing is so interesting? Having managed to keep some of the weight off for several weeks, we concluded that fasting is a fairly effective thing to do, especially if you simply must have a flat stomach in a few days or have an upcoming event that involves a bathing suit. You should not do it for longer than a few days without a doctor and a political cause.

Driving home, we passed Pizza Hut, where they were offering "All-You-Can-Eat for $3.99!"—and we never stopped. Now, *that* was an accomplishment.

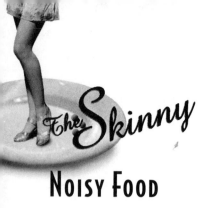

The Skinny

NOISY FOOD

Low calorie = noisy. This occurred to us the other day when we were talking—actually munching—on the phone. How inconvenient, we thought, that nibbling on perfectly fine snacks, like ice or tree bark, happens to sound like road construction work to the person on the other end of the phone. Carrots, celery, radishes, popcorn, melba toast, apples, watermelon—so many foods that are low in calories are also high in fiber and therefore, loud when chewed. Or the high Juice Factor makes them prohibitively rude to eat on the phone—a peach, for instance, needs to be annoyingly slurped. Fattening foods, on the other hand, are mushy and quiet—pudding, ice cream, mashed potatoes, fettuccine Alfredo, Marshmallow Fluff, Velveeta, caramel sauce, cake, chocolate. You can even eat potato chips inconspicuously if you work them over in your mouth long enough.

This is simply an observation, not a tip. We are not suggesting that you eat the Popsicle stick and throw away the Popsicle (though come to think of it, that's not such a bad idea). We realize that you don't need a sound detector to know if something is off-diet-limits. Most likely, you know precisely how many calories are in every item of food available on earth.

Plus, the Noisy Food Theory is admittedly flawed. For instance, think of nuts. We will proceed to another topic before you think of even more exceptions to our scientific principle and tell them to the Nobel Prize on Dieting committee.

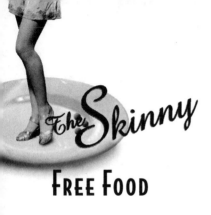

Free Food

There is something inherently evil about free food. It usually tastes pretty good, especially because you didn't cook it or pay for it, and it is usually available in large quantities, and it is almost always something you shouldn't be eating but you find yourself doing it anyway because the price is so good. Free food is the bane of people who want to be skinny. It is the sweet rolls at the breakfast meeting, the shrimp-in-cream-sauce at the luncheon, the lard-laden airplane dinner, the buffet line that never ends. Even radical disciplinarians who haven't had butter in their house in decades see free food and fall apart. Is it thrift that does it? The idea that if the food is free it's also fat-free or calorie-free or just doesn't count because it's . . . out of the ordinary? Is it that free food is usually available in situations when you actually aren't free—you're stuck at a party or trapped in an airplane or something—and eating is one of the only ways to pass the time?

Next time you're offered crème brûlée at no cost, bear in mind these sad facts:

1. Free food is not free in any sense of the word, or in any sense of dieting, or in any sense of reality as we know it.

2. While you are eating it, the freeness of free food is exhilarating. You will eat too much of it. The next day, you will feel doubly awful because you will feel a) fat and b) cheap.

3. When you are about to binge at a buffet, first stop at an ATM and check your bank balance. Less than $100? You probably should eat as much as you can. Anything over $100, you don't need to gorge for survival purposes. Therefore, have a carrot stick and stay at the other side of the room.

4. If you see cat food on sale at rock-bottom prices, do you buy it—even if you don't have a cat? You're the sort of person who should not ever allow yourself to be offered food without a price attached. You are a bargain hunter with no judgment whatsoever. Do not fly, go to parties, attend meetings, go trick-or-treating. Ever.

5. Free coffee is okay, but not if it is accompanied by free donuts, cake, muffins, pancakes, or hot dogs. In that case, it is not free coffee: It is a dark, liquidy gateway drug that will lead you into the abyss. Don't even touch it.

6. Why would you even *want* to eat airplane food? It's awful. You're crazy.

7. Anyway, airplane food isn't really free. You paid something like three dollars for it when you bought your ticket. So if the something-for-nothing part of it appeals to you, take another look at your ticket.

8. Okay, so it's a business trip and someone else paid for your ticket. In which case, return to Tip #6. Why would you even *want* to eat airplane food? It's awful. You're crazy.

9. No one ever gives away free celery sticks. However, if someone ever does, feel free to stuff yourself.

Free Zones

The only temptation more insidious than free food is free food that is in a Free Zone. This is an area within which you believe, on some please-God-let-this-be-true-even-though-I know-better level, that all food has the same calorie and fat content as a stalk of celery; a sort of Twi-lite zone where it is scientifically impossible to get fat. A Free Zone is to a dieter what zero-gravity space might be to a rhinoceros—carte blanche to act uncontrollably insane. Of course, one person's Free Zone is another person's Guilt Belt, but here are some common places of danger:

- the car
- any movie theater
- sidewalks
- airports
- your bed
- the check-out line at the grocery store
- 6 inches in front of an open refrigerator
- children's birthday parties
- other people's plates

If you find yourself losing the Weight War on Free-Zone battlefields, you must change your dieting strategy. Here are some suggestions.

1) Never enter a Free Zone without supervision, even if this means hiring a Nutri-system representative to go to the movies with you.

2) Turn Free Zones into Guilt Belts. We know one woman who keeps a scale in the front seat of her car to remind herself not to stop at a mini-mart along the highway for a hot dog.

3) Stay away from Free Zones altogether. Who says you have to go to the school fair with your children?

4) Engage in activities where it is hard to eat, like bungee jumping. Or hang out at places where food is forbidden:
   - church
   - the dentist's office
   - the operating room at a hospital
   - The Louvre
   - jail
   - under the sea

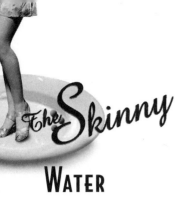

The Skinny

WATER

There's not a diet on the planet that doesn't preach the gospel of eight-glasses-of-water-a-day. And why not respect it? After all, water has the perfect number of calories—zero—and it keeps your mouth busy when you could be eating, say, chocolate mousse, and it's actually even good for you, dieting aside, and sometimes if you drink enough of it water will actually kill your appetite because your stomach is so sodden. We do applaud and recommend water. At the same time, we feel we must tell you the truth, which is: Drinking gallons of water does not make you lose weight. Our nutritional scientist friend gave us the bad news, or we should say, the reality news. Drinking water is just fine, and if you're on a high-protein diet it's especially fine, because your body uses extra water when it is processing protein and you'll feel better if you're not dehydrated. Just don't be fooled into thinking it is miraculously flushing the fat out of your body.

There was a consensus among Skinny Lunch participants that herb tea, which is in our opinion just an alternative form of water, is a dieter's best friend. True, it tastes good, and with a little artificial sweetener you can fool yourself into feeling like you've actually just consumed something desirable, so once again we applaud it—just don't drink it under false pretenses.

If you love seltzer or mineral water, drink up—and then eat very little food, and you will lose weight. If you drink lots and lots of mineral water, check the label. We were once told that in the very fine print of a certain mineral water, there is a barely readable warning that the water contains minute amounts of a Valiumlike substance. We are still looking.

The Skinny

PROTEIN DIETS

This is a not a good time to be a cow. This is not a good time to be a chicken or a lamb or a pig, either. For these days, just about every dieter we know seems to be a carnivore. Protein and fat are good; carbohydrates are bad. Steak and bacon, not to mention cream and cheese are in; pasta and bread and fruit are out.

Many years ago, we were even on protein diets ourselves. Why not? Cheeseburgers are a lot more fun than cooked carrots without butter. And nearly everyone, including us, does seem to lose significant amounts of weight eating all those hefty foods. At least in the beginning.

It is unclear why these diets work. According to the Protein Diet Detractors, these diets take off weight because:

1) Carbohydrates make you retain water whereas protein acts as a diuretic (an effect that stabilizes, they say, after about three weeks).

2) The lack of permissible snack foods—unless you are fond of beef jerky—means you eat less (and less frequently).

3) You end up eating fewer calories per day on these diets because you tend to get sick of eating sooner when you're eating protein than when you're eating carbohydrates.

4) You lose your appetite because of nausea. Detractors also say that these diets can be horribly dangerous if you go on them for a long, long time; but, come on, who's going to go on any diet for a long, long time?

Protein Diet Enthusiasts talk a lot about the Eskimos, a fit and healthy group who eat almost no carbohydrates. They also talk a lot about body chemistry. The theory behind low-carbohydrate, high-protein diets, in a nutshell (nuts are allowed), is this: The easiest and most common way for your body to get energy is through glucose which comes from carbohydrates. The more glucose you produce, the higher your insulin level. Insulin is bad because it encourages the storage of fat. On the other hand, when you deprive your body of carbs by eating mostly protein and fat, you must instead draw on your own fat for energy. And anything that eats away at your own fat is something to be cheered.

If you like steak and butter, you should probably try this diet, at least for a week or two. It has worked for many women and it may well work for you. But don't count on eating all the mayonnaise and macadamia nuts you want. It doesn't work that way.

The Skinny

Ripe Fruit vs. Nonripe Fruit

Only a highly neurotic dieter would decide that ripe fruit, because it is sweeter than unripe fruit, therefore contains more calories. But we know our audience. And you happen to be correct. What happens with age (the age of the fruit, not yours) is that some nondigestible fiber is broken down into digestible molecules. The difference is slight, but slight to one person is robust to another. And it is not only a question of calories, according to some nutritionists. As a fruit ripens, the starch breaks down into simpler sugars which create more blood sugar. In the case of the banana, for instance, the process of ripening increases the blood sugar by 70% (writes Philip Lipetz in *The Good Calorie Count,* and he took it from K. Hermansen et al. in *Diabetic Medicine* 9, 1992, and T.M.S. Wolever et al. in *J. Clin. Nutr. Gastroenterol.* 3, 1988 . . . if you want to get term-paper-y about it). If you are someone who cares about blood sugar, and not everybody does, avoid ripe bananas.

Then again, it is unclear why you would go for the green, unripe banana. Of course, you could put NutraSweet on it until it is sweet enough to enjoy. But then you're up to just about the same calorie count as ripe fruit. For what it's worth, here are the comparisons between an unripe apple and a ripe one.

APPLE		
SIZE	FRESH	RIPE
	NUMBER OF CALORIES	NUMBER OF CALORIES
Small 2.5 in. dia.	59	63
Med. small 2.75 in. dia.	77	83
Med. large 3 in. dia.	93	99
Large 3.25 in. dia.	118	127

The Outside vs. the Inside of Food

Are you an outsider or an insider? No, we are not exploring your alienation from society; nor are we curious about the direction of your belly button. We are talking about whether you prefer the inside or outside of food. During Skinny Lunches we noticed that many women picked at their rolls, eating only the crust or pinches of dough; or they pulled the skin off their chicken; or scraped the icing off cake.

If you do have such bizarre leanings—even if you are eclectic and like the inside of some foods and the outside of others—you are lucky. Here's why: 1) As we learned in first grade, a fraction of a whole is always less than the whole. Therefore, when it comes to food, it is always better to like part of something than the whole. A better way to state this: It is always better to dislike part of something than like the whole thing and the bigger the part you dislike, the better. 2) Peeling, shucking, and skinning food requires work; and work takes time; and time lowers the Calories Per Minute of a food (see The Skinny on Calories Per Minute). You may even get so fed up trying to separate the inside from the outside, that you'll leave the dinner table before you take a bite. We doubt it, though. 3) If you limit yourself to either the outside or the inside of food, you will run out of stuff to eat sooner than if you'll eat just any old thing.

Egg, large
White	16 calories
Yolk	63 calories

Chicken
Skin, 1 oz	129 calories
White meat, 4 oz	196 calories
Dark meat, 4 oz	232 calories

Baked potato
Skin, 2 oz	75 calories
Inside, 4 oz	105 calories

Chocolate cupcake
Cake	103 calories
Chocolate frosting	72 calories

Apple (medium
3 in. diameter)
Without skin	82 calories
Skin	11 calories

Bread

inside = outside (the outside may be brushed with oil or butter but the difference in calories is infinitesimal)

Oreo

Unfortunately, we are unable to give you a calorie count of the cream filling vs. the chocolate wafer. According to the woman in customer relations at Nabisco, a lot of people call the 800 number asking for this information, but "the kitchen just won't give us that breakdown." What are they afraid of?

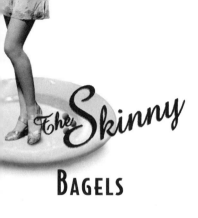

The Skinny

BAGELS

By any chance have you ever heard of . . . *Satan*???

Okay, maybe not Satan, but not the Good Fairy of Food Products, either. Yes, bagels are fat-free (until you plaster on the cream cheese, at least) but they are calorie- and carbo-dense. Try weighing one sometime. A typical bagel weighs about, oh, 5 pounds, and (seriously) might have as many as 600 calories. Two bagels and you've eaten your daily ration of calories, practically, even if you think you've just had a little post-workout snack.

If you can't live without bagels, what are your options? Always get plain—sesame seeds and poppy seeds have calories, after all. Always get a bialy instead of a bagel, if you have the option—they have half as many calories and are almost as good. The truly skinny split their bagels in thirds and throw away the middle third, which doesn't have any of the good chewy crust, anyway, so it's no great loss (except in calories). The really, really skinny then scoop out the insides. This leaves the shape and essential character of the bagel, but mostly just crust, and a lot fewer calories.

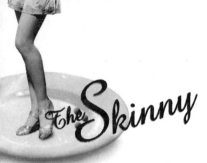

The Skinny

Comparing Apples and Oranges

Apple	82 calories
Orange	65 calories

The Skinny

ARTIFICIAL SWEETENERS

Once upon a time, there were no such things as artificial sweeteners. Sweet things tasted sweet because they contained sugar or honey or molasses, and they had calorie counts that reflected their sweetness (770 calories per cup of sugar, 60 calories per tablespoon of honey, 70 calories per tablespoon of molasses). Then along came saccharin and aspartame—Sweet'n Low and NutraSweet to you—and suddenly you could slam down a six-pack of teeth-grindingly sweet diet Coke and not be a calorie richer for it. Heaven! Or so it seems, except for the fact that saccharin afflicted lab rats with bladder cancer and brain dysfunction and aspartame, some claim, imparts headaches, epilepsy, memory loss, nausea, and depression. News like that makes us so upset that the only thing that will console us is a Sugar-free Fat-free Fudgsicle and a handful of Extra-Strength Excedrin. Can't we ever win? Can't we have our Equal and our brain cells too?

What's worse, some scientists insist that the taste of anything sweet—whether it's the real thing or artificial—triggers the release of insulin into the bloodstream, which causes an increase in your appetite. In other words, you may be getting off easy with your zero-calorie diet Coke, but according to these studies, you'll just end up ravenous and probably will eventually give in to a piece of chocolate cheesecake. Another study argues that aspartame blocks the production of serotonin, which your body manufactures to regulate appetite and elevate mood. In other words, too much sugar-free Jell-O might make you hungry and depressed, our top two most unfavorite sensations.

Like all cold, hard, scientific data, there are just as many studies (probably financed by the NutraSweet Company of America, but remember, these science things are expensive) that say artificial sweeteners 1) don't make you hungry; 2) can't possibly block enough serotonin to make a significant difference in your mood; and 3) are a true blessing for fat people—and, for that matter, normal-sized people who don't necessarily want to ingest a million calories every time they have a yen for something sweet.

We're all over the map with this one. First of all, we both consume large (huge) quantities of artificial sweeteners, so much that no laboratory rat will get near us for fear of breathing in our toxicity. Still, as of this writing, we appear to be brain-intact, which is no guarantee for the future, but then again, there are no guarantees in the future. (Note: We are still brain-active enough to have a lively disagreement on which artificial sweetener we love the most—Susan swears by Equal, Patty likes to use a combination of sweeteners.) We use sweeteners liberally and maintain that they can turn almost any tasteless substance (cottage cheese, shaved ice, herbal tea) into a decent dessert substitute with a very minimal weight impact, as long as you don't heat it (NutraSweet at least seems to lose its taste when heated). How could that possibly be depressing? On the other hand, we have both noticed that the less sweet stuff we eat (real or artificial), the less we seem to want. Then again, the only times we don't want sweet stuff are times when we don't really want anything to eat at all, so it's hard to distinguish between cause and effect. As quantity eaters, we worry that the philosophy of "have a bit of the real thing, it'll be more satisfying and you'll be happy with just a smidge" doesn't apply to us. Just a smidge of flourless chocolate cake? Why not the whole cake? If it's so damn good, why would you be happy with just a smidge?

Which is why, finally, we are committed fakers. When we're craving sweets, we're craving a lot of sweets, and we might as well try to contain the damage by making them fake sweets. True, there is that false sense of security when you're eating fake things—the kind of security that leads you to eat entire boxes of fat-free cookies rather than a civilized one or two. To avert that, we just ruin our appetite midway through our binge by thinking: They say it's sugar-free and calorie-free, but maybe they're lying. . . . Amazing how you suddenly don't want to eat more.

This might all change with the recent introduction of a new sugar substitute called "stevia," an herbal powder that is much sweeter than aspartame, is all-natural and allegedly harmless. This would get rid of the brain damage aspects of today's artificial sweeteners, but it wouldn't necessarily change the sweet-tooth problem, that tasting sweetness will make you hungrier regardless of what the sweetness is. Of course, we can always dream.

THIS JUST IN: The executive committee of the

157

National Toxicology Program, a government advisory health group, voted in December 1998 to give saccharin a clean bill of health. To this, we say "Drink up!"

WHAT TO PUT ARTIFICIAL SWEETENER ON

Celery

Already-sweetened iced tea

Cottage cheese

Rice (and you have rice pudding!)

Plain pasta (and you have noodle pudding!)

Egg white omelettes (*voilà* . . . dessert crepes!)

Pencil tips

All fruit except watermelon (on second thought, Nutra-watermelon sounds tasty)

Raisins (a treat to watch movies by)

WHAT NOT TO PUT ARTIFICIAL SWEETENER ON

Meat

Diet Coke

Hard liquor

Pizza

Halibut

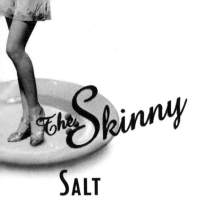

The Skinny

SALT

Salt does not make you fat. Don't worry about it. (The day after eating a soy-sauce-heavy Chinese dinner your rings will feel tight. This will go away after an hour or two. If your rings feel tight and you didn't have Chinese food anytime recently, you probably are fat and it has nothing to do with salt and you should eat less food of all kinds, including Chinese.)

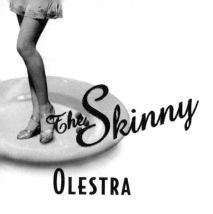

OLESTRA

Strictly for research purposes, we tried a no-fat
WOW potato chip, made with olestra (the new nonfat
fat that passes through the body undigested) and containing half the calories of regular potato chips (75
calories an ounce). We have eaten them nonstop ever
since. They are too salty and have a slightly stale
taste, but we kind of like the taste of staleness. The
problem is not that they make you sick if you eat too
many, which it is impossible not to do. (Loose stools is
how they describe it on the package, and that is fairly
accurate.) The problem is not that they may cause
liver damage at the worst or deplete you of essential
nutrients at best—though some scientists say that is
nonsense, though many of those scientists happen to
work for Frito-Lay, who make *WOW* potato chips, or
Procter & Gamble, who make *Olean,* the brand name
for olestra. The problem is that we never ate potato
chips before we tried *WOW* potato chips. Potato
chips were taboo. As were *Doritos, Ruffles,* and
Pringles which also come with olestra and also have
that stale taste we have grown fond of. So, while it is
nice that *WOW* potato chips are only 75 calories instead of 150 calories an ounce and no grams of fat in-

stead of 10 grams of fat, it remains that we were eating zero calories and zero grams of fat of potato chips before Procter & Gamble came up with olestra.

A note to Frito-Lay: Please do not invent fat-free cheese doodles.

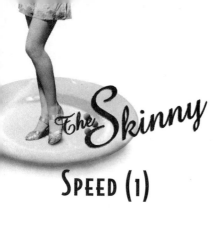

The Skinny

SPEED (1)

Ah, ephedrine! The dieter's elixir. It kills the appetite and increases metabolism. Women drop pounds in days without changing their eating or exercise habits. Muscle mass, which is usually the first to go on fad diets, is spared when weight is lost the ephedrine way. Combined with caffeine and aspirin—as it is in many weight-loss pills, powders, and teas—the potency of the drug rises exponentially. Often, herbal laxatives and diuretics are also thrown into the mix for added oomph.

Products containing ephedrine or members of its chemical family are sold in health food stores and over the Internet. *Cybergenics, Quick Trim, Black Cross, Metabolift, Ultra Diet Pep, Eph 833,* and *Ripped Fuel* are just a few. Ephedrine is the magical ingredient in *Herbal Ecstasy,* which is the "natural" form of the drug MDMA (4-methyl-2-dimethoxyamphetamine, technically). The brand names give you a pretty good idea as to the drug's promise: *Cloud 9, Herbal Ecstasy,* and *Ultimate Xphoria.* Ephedrine's botanical version, Chinese *ma huang* or *ephedra sinica,* is sometimes known as "legal speed." Ephedrine is also related to pseudoephedrine, the drug that gives nasal decongestants like Sudafed its zip and Comtrex its zing. Indeed, at a

Skinny Lunch during which we asked everyone to name her #1 diet tip, one woman dug into her tote bag and simply held up Tylenol Sinus.

Ephedrine does not just melt fat and transform you into the happiest person alive. Athletic performance can be enhanced and sexual awareness heightened. Compared to all that, safety seems like a trivial concern. We don't want to be irresponsible, though. (Okay, we do; but we know better.) Is it dangerous? Depends whom you ask. According to even its supporters, ephedrine may cause dry mouth, nervousness, nauseousness, headaches, gastrointestinal distress, insomnia, inability to concentrate, and heart palpitations—and those are the *good* bad side effects. The *bad* bad side effects include psychosis, psychological and/or physiological addiction, heart arrythmias, paranoia, stroke, and ventricular fibrillation. The very worst side effect is death. The FDA is trying to regulate herbal forms of ephedrine, and in the meantime, has urged people not to use these products. They are already illegal in seventeen states.

Boosters of ephedrine, however, argue that only a fractional percentage of people are "intolerant" to the drug. They agree that it should not be used if you have heart problems, angina, hypertension, thyroid problems, or an enlarged prostate, but they insist that nearly all deaths related to ephedrine have been caused by overdoses. They remind us that juice made from ephedra has been available in China for 5,200 years—of course, so has poison. . . .

We know lots of people who have lost weight taking ephedrine. They are all alive, though one did faint.

SPEED (2)

Skinny women don't eat like puppies, lapping up everything on the plate. They eat slowly, sometimes painfully slowly. Sometimes it is so frustrating to watch a slow eater eat, you want to jump up from the table and cram the food down her throat. But that's the risk a slow eater takes in order to be skinny. And so should you. Here's how to become one of Them:

- At a restaurant, be the one to talk, not listen. Listeners eat too much.
- Eat with silverware and a plate. Equipment slows you down.
- Cut your food into tiny pieces. This also slows you down.
- Chew and chew and chew and chew.
- Let everyone else use the salt and pepper before you do. If you are the last to start eating and you keep to a slow eating pace, you will eat less.
- At a dinner party, offer to clear the plates. Otherwise you'll sit there and, well, clear the food.
- Don't eat as if you are in a Sam Shepard play—stool in front of the open refrigerator, feet up on the counter, take-out Chinese container in your

grubby hands. This encourages high-velocity eating.

- Remember that this isn't the last time you are going to eat. Food will always be available. (And if it's not, good!)
- Play with your food, if you must, to keep from eating when you're not hungry. How tall a "french fries log cabin" can you stack on your plate?
- Pause every so often during a meal. This will not only lower your CPM (see The Skinny on Calories Per Minute), but it will help you figure out whether you're eating out of hunger or momentum.

The Skinny

DRINKING

We all know fat alcoholics and we all know thin alcoholics. For legal reasons, we cannot name names. Besides, gossip, while fun, isn't really the point. We are here to discuss the effect that drinking has on weight. Two questions are pertinent.

• Does being sloshed make you eat more or less? Most research indicates that drinking causes you to eat more (partly because your body does not "notice" the calories that come from alcohol and so you remain hungry). And not only more, but worse. It is the rare and lucky drunk who has a few martinis and then proceeds to eat carrots and nonfat yogurt uncontrollably. On the contrary, studies show that being crocked makes you crave protein—lots and lots of the fattening kind. That said, a sizable minority of Skinny Lunchers claimed that alcohol caused them to lose interest in food. One woman told us that she drank a glass of wine after dinner as a dessert surrogate. Cheers to you, too, if you can manage to drink moderately without ordering everything on the menu (conking out helps).

• Does drinking alter your metabolism? Yes, but the way in which it does so depends on how much alcohol you drink. If you drink a moderate amount of liquor, your body will burn fat slower. In other words, you will put on weight. But become a rip-roaring drunk and your body will learn how to "waste" the calories that come from alcohol. The 7 calories a gram that alcohol ordinarily provides will not be stored as 7 calories of fat. This metabolic inefficiency was the basis of the Drinking Man's Diet, the popular 1960s diet which recommended substituting alcohol for sugars and starches. Unfortunately, the same process that enables a serious drinker's body to dissipate alcohol's calories as useless heat also creates a lot of dangerous chemicals in your body that can indirectly lead to diseases you don't want, like cirrhosis of the liver and cancer of the esophagus. You'll be skinny, but dead skinny.

Though we've just explained why calories are not always important when it comes to alcohol, we can't help but be interested in a comparative calorie count of various types of booze. And so:

	CALORIES PER OUNCE
Chablis	22
Champagne	25
Soave	27
Dry sherry	36
Campari	47
Distilled spirits, 80 proof	65
Distilled spirits, 90 proof	75
Distilled spirits, 100 proof	85
Amaretto	80

Drambuie	110
Tia Maria	92
Light beer	8
Regular beer	12 (dark beers have more calories than lighter lagers)

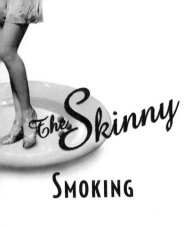

SMOKING

The Surgeon General is not going to be happy with this, but it's true: Smoking tends to be an appetite suppressant, decreasing the desire for simple carbohydrates (sweets). It also inhibits the efficiency with which food is metabolized. Indeed, just consuming nicotine burns calories, which made us wonder if we would lose weight wearing a nicotine patch or chewing nicotine gum. Sadly, though, little research has been done in this area. And, oh—there's some evidence that smoking may forestall the symptoms of Alzheimer's disease, but that's someone else's book.

Many skinny women have spent their happiest and sveltest days smoking. Most we know have quit altogether, although a few still smoke a couple cigarettes a day, claiming that it really helps to keep their weight down. One smoker told us she takes a smoking break during a meal to curb her appetite. Those who have quit often still dream of cigarettes—one wannabe smoker told us that her ideal food would be deep fried cigarettes rolled in sugar. Smoking is a sport among models.

Then there's the bad news. In case you have just spent your entire life in a coma, we must break it to you that smoking is not healthy. It causes lots of diseases, many of them fatal (although you usually do end up thin). We are not recommending smoking. We would get in too much trouble for that. Neither of us has ever smoked, although Patty once considered going to Smoke Starters to take off a couple pounds. We want to simply point out that if living is not one of your goals, smoking might be the weight-loss approach for you.

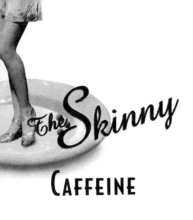

The Skinny

CAFFEINE

Next time someone tells you how unhealthy caffeine is, point out that there are fewer suicides among those who drink coffee than those who don't. We wonder if that's because they're thinner. Though most scientists swear caffeine isn't an appetite suppressant and that it affects metabolism only marginally, it is also true that caffeine is a diuretic. In fact, because caffeine, applied topically, draws water from fat cells, it gives your skin a less-dimpled look. This is why it is a chief ingredient in many expensive anti-cellulite creams. (You can save a lot of money by simply massaging the used—and warm—coffee grounds from your coffee machine onto your cellulite-afflicted body parts.)

But regardless of what scientists say, we know from experience that drinking vats of diet Coke, coffee, and iced tea makes us so wired we RUNAND-JUMPANDFIDGETANDFORGETABOUT-FOOD!!

THE FRENCH QUESTION

Why do French women look so incredible? This question came up again and again at the Skinny Lunches, along with the observation that it just isn't fair. The French break every diet rule: They consume vast quantities of bread, cheese, and wine. They pour sauce on everything that is not alive (the only time they refrain from using butter is when they use cream). And they never exercise unless you count lighting cigarettes.

Naturally, we were too jealous ever to invite a French woman to a Skinny Lunch, but we did include an Italian woman, an Australian woman, and a woman who had lived in Canada for a few years. The latter told us that when she was a teenager her friend swore to her that French women had great bodies because French bread had no calories.

We looked into several other theories. *Are French men more attractive than American men, thus providing women more of an incentive to stay in shape and become mistresses?* Not necessarily—remember Charles de Gaulle? *Do foie gras and béchamel sauce contain secret slimming ingredients when made in France?* No, according to a woman who had gained a lot of weight in France eating only foie gras and béchamel sauce.

Perhaps the deconstructionist Jacques Derrida knows some-thing about the breakup of fat cells that we don't know? Uh, we're saving Derrida's book for the beach this summer. *What about all that nude sunbathing in France?* What about it?

After lengthy discussion, we decided that the reason French women look better than we do has partly to do with their clothes and mostly to do with their eating habits. They do not eat pizza, hot dogs, and ice cream on the street—at least not all at once. They don't consider television a form of cheap dinner theater during which you try to shovel as much food as you can into your mouth before you fall asleep in your recliner. Finally, the All-You-Can-Eat concept has yet to hit France, a country where restaurants still serve portions that actually fit on a plate.

But just wait. The French are beginning to eat like the Americans. Packaged cereal and hot chocolate made from mix are replacing bakery-fresh bread and coffee as the typical French breakfast. McDonald's has become a popular family restaurant in Paris. Coca-Cola is replacing water or fruit-flavored water as the favorite drink among children. Obesity is now 8 percent among the French population and on the rise. Soon there will be a Sara Lee cheesecake in every French refrigerator and a Dunkin' Donuts on every rue. America will spoil the dainty French figure. It is only a matter of time. And we're looking forward to it!

The Skinny

How to Look
Skinny in a Photo
(If You're Not Skinny)

Photos lie, so we might as well have them lie in our favor. This requires some groundwork. That is, stand on the ground next to an elephant so that you will look delicate and petite in juxtaposition. If this isn't possible, then at least you can make sure you are not wearing clothes that feature a big pattern or plaid. Horizontal stripes are not desirable, unless they are on the elephant. If a wide-angle lens is being used, stand in the middle. Anyone on an end will appear stretched-out horizontally, never a good look unless you are lying down.

Lighting is essential. Make that, lack of lighting. In general, the darker, the better. (Come on, why do you think all those people really choose to be interviewed on *60 Minutes* in shadow?) If you do not have control over lights and shadows (and truly only God does), you can compensate with your makeup. Your makeup should make you look angular, but with big lips and big eyes. Use Munch's *The Scream* as your model. Darken the area under the chin and apply a scumbled dark line under the cheekbones even if you don't have cheekbones. Your hair should elongate your face. No bangs (unless you have other factors besides skinniness to consider).

Now for the pose. Hands on hips so there's a space between your arms and your body. Shoulders back. Chin down. Cheeks sucked in. Lips pursed. Eyes coquettishly up in a doelike gaze. And don't ruin it by saying cheese. It's fattening in more ways than one.

If you've been caught off guard by the camera, don't worry. The most important part of the photo is still to come. The Retouch.

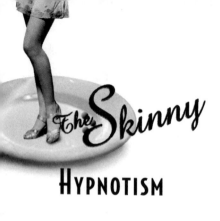

The Skinny

HYPNOTISM

A while ago, we were looking for a technique that would stop us from occasionally eating, oh, say, approximately five hundred times the normal quantity. (See The Skinny on Quantity vs. Quality.) Hypnosis seemed the perfect solution. It was fast, it supposedly curbs irrational behavior, and it seems to promise that thing we all want: magic. Hypnosis has been used to treat everything from fear of going to the dentist to plantar warts to poison ivy. Basically, it works by drawing someone into a state so unguarded that she is made extraordinarily susceptible to the power of suggestion.

On the basis of the Eye Test, Susan was a better candidate for hypnosis than Patty. The Eye Test? Keep your head level and roll your eyes upward. The more white area that shows, the better the chance that you can be hypnotized. Susan's eyes reveal such a scary amount of white, she is probably also a good candidate for being put into a coma. The insufficiency of white in Patty's eyes, on the other hand, indicates she might have trouble following even simple directions like "Turn left," let alone hypnotic suggestions. Nevertheless, she, like Susan, hoped that on the way home from the first session with hypnotist Julie Flanders, she would mysteriously drop 20 pounds instantly.

During the first of our four sessions ($100 each), Julie emphasized talk therapy more than we'd expected. While we weren't initially curious about what circumstances were conducive to our eating like maniacs, it was, admittedly interesting, and in a subtle way, helpful. During each session, Julie talked us into a trance, soothingly guiding us through relaxation exercises (which is another way of saying, droning on until you are so bored, you almost fall asleep). While we were in a hypnotic state, Julie intoned about positive body images and moderate eating habits, often referencing specific examples from our lives we had talked about with her earlier. Julie gave us tapes of the session which we were supposed to listen to every day. We promptly lost the tapes. (A skinny friend of ours who had been to a hypnotist described what was on her tape: "In this world of commas and dots, I have a feeling that you, Elizabeth, are an exclamation point! Are you going to succumb to the cookie? Who's stronger—you or the cookie? . . ."

After the first session, we walked home, eating everything in sight along the way. We wondered if Julie had misunderstood our goal and instilled within us the urge to pig out. By the second session, though, we had stopped overeating. In fact, aside from that caloric walk home the first day, we have not binged since we met Julie. Though we did not lose weight, hypnotism does seem a fairly effective way to deal with automatic, mindless eating.

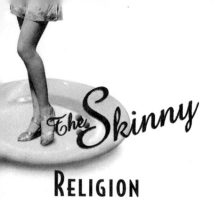

RELIGION

A lot of people have died in the name of religion, but according to Gwen Shamblin in *The Weigh Down Diet* (1997), you can diet in the name of religion, too. He—as in HE—can teach you how never to overeat. He can fill you with that same blissful feeling you get from food but with none of the "yucky, guilty, depressing side effects." He can lead you not into the temptation of chips and dip. The *Weigh Down Diet* was a big seller, but maybe that's because the only exercise it exhorted was "getting down on your knees to pray. . . ."

At the risk of being struck down fat, we must report that a study by researchers at Purdue University found that religious people in the United States are more likely than nonreligious people to be overweight. In light of this, it's hard to agree with Gwen Shamblin that God is "the genius of behavior modification." However, we do agree that religion can be skinny-friendly:

- Religion develops your guilt skills.
- Most religions include at least one fast a year.
- The superreligious can observe a fat-free Lent or bread-free Passover year-round.

- There is never even one thing you want to eat at Potluck Suppers.
- Most religions either forbid alcohol or limit the amount and time you can drink, with the exception of the Episcopalians.
- What if we told you that admission to Heaven was based on how much you weigh?

Oh, by the way. A communion wafer is 5 calories tops. But don't go ruining it by drinking too much wine.

WHY YOU SHOULD NEVER TELL YOUR MOTHER YOU'RE ON A DIET

If you think you have a distorted body image, wait until you ask your mother to describe you. In her eyes, you are either perfect or you are . . . let's just say, the opposite of perfect. Which is why you should never let your mother know you have ever had the slightest thought about your weight, let alone desperately want to change it. Should you be overcome by temporary insanity, however, and mention to your mother that you are trying to slim down a bit, be prepared to hear one or several of the following:

1) "I know you just started the diet an hour ago, but how much weight have you lost so far?"

2) "Good idea. Let's go on a diet together. I'll race you."

3) "Why would you want to change yourself? You are so beautiful. And if you just stood up straight, pushed your hair out of your eyes, wore some less drab clothes, bleached your teeth, got contact lenses (preferably tinted), bought a rug for your living room,

and changed your personality, you would probably be married in a week."

4) "I knew it! You're anorexic. I can tell just by listening to your voice on the phone-answering machine that you need to be hospitalized."

5) "As a matter of fact, I have noticed in excruciating detail and discussed at length with my friends and your friends and your siblings and most of our relatives and people you don't even know that you've been looking a little chunky lately, but honey, I'm your mother and you know I love you no matter how chunky you are."

6) "Darling, I think you look perfectly adorable in those huge, shapeless tunics and sacklike drawstring-waist pants. It reminds me of when you were my chubby little adorable baby! You were so cute!"

7) "Who told you to lose weight?"

8) "Only five pounds?"

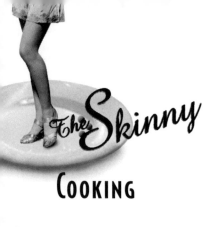

The Skinny

COOKING

Unless you have a generous expense account or feel you can exist on a diet of raw hot dogs and chewing gum, you'll probably have to cook now and then. Lucky you! Seriously! You're lucky because when you cook for yourself you can cook what you want, the way you want it, and never have to be haunted by questions like "Is this silky soup base really nonfat yogurt or is it, in fact, two full pints of heavy cream?" If you made the silky soup base yourself, you'd know. Knowledge is both fat-free and powerful.

Cooking skinnily isn't hard. The cardinal rules are as follows:

1. Play rough with recipes. If something calls for a cup of oil, try making it with only half a cup. Or a quarter cup. Or no oil at all. Usually you won't even miss it.

2. Cut the amount of butter called for by half or more (we usually leave it out altogether).

3. Steam or poach things instead of browning or frying them, especially if they're only secondary ingredients. Granted, they may not be quite as delicious, but look at it this way: If they're not as delicious, you

won't eat as much, which is another diet plus. Honestly, if you're making chicken with some kind of sauce, why not steam or poach the chicken (fat-free) rather than browning it in oil? It's the sauce you're going to end up tasting anyway, and you'll save a lot of calories painlessly.

4. Leave out fattening ingredients like nuts, avocados, cheese, raisins, and olives. If you feel you absolutely can't live without them, sprinkle them on at the last minute, like a garnish. This will trick you into thinking you are eating more than you actually are. Ingredients cooked together tend to meld together; anything put in at the last minute like a garnish will stand out. Often the flavor of these fattening taste treats will stand out so much more when added late that you won't mind having only a tiny amount. For instance, if you love dressing your salad with olive oil, try first dousing it with lemon juice and/or balsamic vinegar and/or salt and pepper and/or fat-free dressing. Then drizzle on a smidgen of olive oil—make sure you get really good olive oil, which has a lot of flavor, rather than the IGA House Brand or anything marked "Armed Forces Surplus." You'll smell the oil and taste it and probably won't notice how little you've actually put on.

If you have a recipe that uses nuts, particularly in a topping (some kind of baked fish with pecan topping or even apple crisp), try substituting toasted breadcrumbs—the toasting makes them taste nutty, and the texture is close. Another good nut substitute is Grape-Nuts cereal, which is not nuts at all and is fat-free and very crunchy.

5. Make friends with Pam. Or Misto. Or any of

those cooking sprays, which can cut way down on your cooking oil and really does get things browned up pretty nicely.

6. Also, make friends with Teflon. Crummy nonstick cookware makes everything seem sort of rubbery, but good nonstick pans are terrific when you're trying to brown food without using a ton of oil. The way to know if it's good is if it's expensive. Our favorite nonstick pan technique is to spray Pam (olive oil flavor) on a medium hot Le Creuset nonstick skillet, slap down a skinless chicken breast, let it sizzle away until it's good and toasty, flip it and let the other side get brown, and then turn the heat down so the inside of the chicken gets cooked through. If the outside of the chicken is getting too burned, sprinkle a little bit of water or wine or vinegar into the pan, just to release some steam, and also so you can scrape up the burned bits from the bottom of the pan (very tasty pan juice, we might add). We advise keeping your kitchen window open and your exhaust fan on High whenever you're cooking this way, because things do tend to burn when you're not lubricating them with lots of oil.

7. If something is roastable, then roast it. A good cookbook for this is Barbara Kafka's *Roasting,* which tells you how to heat-blast just about anything. She's reasonably light-handed with the oil, but you can use even a little less than she suggests. Almost everything tastes really good if it's roasted, even without any oil at all.

8. Better yet, take everything out into the backyard and barbecue it.

9. Get skinny cooking equipment. It will make you feel good, even if you don't use it that much. For in-

stance, if you're serious about losing weight, you shouldn't be eating a lot of gravy, but you might as well have a gravy skimmer anyway for those occasional gravy moments. A skimmer is a pitcher that miraculously and magically separates the grease from the gravy, and it'll cost only a few bucks.

Another indispensable is an indoor grill. The one we love is the George Foreman Lean Mean Grilling Machine, a weird-looking electric device that is kind of a giant waffle iron set at an angle. You place the food product—fish fillet, vegetable, chicken breast—on the grill surface, close the cover, watch as the grease drips out the angled bottom, and in about two minutes your food is cooked. It's great; it requires no oil; it makes authentic-looking grill marks on the food, which makes you feel you're having a wonderful picnic rather than some dried-up tasteless diet meal. There are other indoor electric countertop grills which are undoubtedly good, but the George Foreman's special asset is the way it sits at an angle, which helps degrease even grease-intense items like pork chops.

We've also tried out those Korean water barbecues. They're ring-shaped pans that you fill with water and place on your stovetop, then cover with a grill surface that's usually nonstick. The food is steam/grilled, which works very well with thin, sticky things like fish and meat, but less well with vegetables (they seem to roll around too much and don't cook through). Overall, it's a mixed blessing, but worth trying.

10. Never underestimate lemon juice, wine, and vinegar. These are nearly calorie-free and totally fat-free elixirs that work on fish, chicken, meat, vegetables, starches—and can be used to moisten and unstick practically everything.

11. For that matter, never underestimate the miracle of fat-free plain yogurt. You can't exactly cook with it (it'll separate when heated up) but you can add it to anything to create the illusion of creaminess—soup, mashed potatoes, spreads, salad dressing.

12. Stock up on mustard, chutney, spices, and herbs, and use liberally to take your mind off the relative blandness of your low-calorie food. Poached chicken breast will always depress you if you're dieting. However, chicken breast that is coated with something like a) exotic mustard or b) crushed pepper or c) a mixture of cumin and coriander, and then grilled (preferably on the George Foreman or its equivalent) actually tastes like food a real person might desire.

13. If a recipe calls for chicken with skin, ignore it and take the skin off anyway. It rarely makes a difference.

14. You can substitute turkey for almost everything and save a zillion calories. Use ground turkey in chili, turkey breast in stews, smoked turkey instead of ham, turkey sausage instead of pepperoni. Chicken is okay, too, but turkey is leaner and tastes meatier.

15. Buy lots of low-fat cookbooks. Once you get the hang of it, start tweaking those recipes, too—they're good but still usually include the requisite good-sense, all-is-moderation amounts of fat, and since we do not advocate good sense and moderation, we say to hell with it—if you're going to make something low-fat, how about no-fat?

16. If a recipe calls for foie gras, don't make it.

17. Never, ever, ever deep-fry anything, even for a second.

18. Anytime you can use a vegetable instead of a

starch, try it. Spaghetti squash can be a great (and much lower-calorie) pasta. It does sound improbable, but when it's cooked, spaghetti squash turns into little strings that do a convincing imitation of linguine for about one-tenth of the calories, and tastes fine with any pasta sauce. Eggplant can be sliced like loaves of bread and used as pizza crust—before you gag, remember that a whole eggplant is only 90 calories, while a real pizza crust is several million. It's probably even healthy for you (not that we're promoting that or anything—it's just an interesting fact).

19. Fat-free salad dressing is a dieter's helper—not just to use with salad, but also as an oil substitute in certain recipes. If you're making pesto, for instance, try blending the basil and garlic with fat-free Italian dressing instead of olive oil (or just add a drizzle of oil). We also leave out the delicious but nastily fattening Parmesan cheese. The result is not exactly the same as traditional pesto, but it's good. Some fat-free dressings are just awful, so shop carefully. We like a brand called Annie's, which seems to be widely distributed. If the dressing is good enough, it can even work as a guilt-free sauce; Annie's Fat-Free Dijon-Honey Dressing is great on chicken, and Wish-Bone Fat Free Blue Cheese Dressing is good on baked potatoes.

20. If a recipe calls for a lot of cheese, don't make it. If it calls for a little bit of cheese, use even less and make sure it's strong-flavored—Roquefort or good-quality Parmigiana-Reggiano—so you'll taste it even if you use microscopic amounts. Skim-milk mozzarella and fat-free goat cheese are practically indistinguishable from the real thing, but most other fat-free cheese is not very good, so use with caution. Replac-

ing aged Vermont cheddar in a recipe with Joe's Lo-lo No-flava Chedda is likely to disappoint. Better to find something else to cook.

21. If you feel that life isn't worth living if you can't have chicken-fried steak, try bake-frying: Dredge the chicken/eggplant/fish in flour, dip it in lightly beaten egg whites and then in fine bread crumbs. Place in a nonstick pan that has been sprayed with oil. Bake in a hot oven—400 degrees—for 30 to 45 minutes (adjust cooking time for the type of food). To make it really good, season the flour with savory spices like paprika, ground pepper, garlic powder, sage, or marjoram.

22. Another nonbutter, noncream way to thicken sauces, soups, etc., is by adding a small amount of pureed white cannellini beans (use the canned ones; don't bother making them from scratch, obviously). The beans have a fairly neutral taste and are fat-free.

DO NOT APPLY THE PREVIOUS RULES TO BAKING

The physics of baked goods are trickier than the physics of, say, beef stew. Beef stew can be thickened, thinned, watered down, and beefed up to your heart's content, but you can't mess around with baked goods quite as liberally. Cookie dough made with all the butter left out, for instance, is not going to turn into cookies, and if you tinker too much with recipes for things that have to rise, you may find them either deflating or exploding. There are tricks for skinnifying baked goods but you can't modify most recipes wholesale—you've got to do proper substitutions or you'll end up with a mess.

1. Skip the egg yolks. Or at least, minimize them. You can usually substitute two egg whites for one egg yolk. If a recipe calls for four yolks, try using just one or two (for color and taste) and then egg whites for the rest.

2. Experiment, cautiously, with fat replacements. It works best if what you're experimenting with is not absolutely crucial to the edibility and texture of the dish; for instance, we've had great success making fat-free apple crisp by replacing the butter with fat-free yogurt because the main part of the dish is the apples; the butter is just used to make the topping taste good, and the yogurt is a fair substitute. Anyway, apple crisp is just an excuse for eating warm apples topped with sugar, so who cares if the topping is a little mushy? It still tastes good.

3. Nuts are delicious but oh-so-fattening. You won't miss them if you leave them out of things like chocolate-chip cookies, which you shouldn't be eating anyway but if you feel you must, you can at least be a little disciplined and skip the walnuts (roughly 700 calories for 4 ounces. See what we mean?)

4. There is no way to make pastry dough and pie crusts without using a ton of butter, so you might as well forget it.

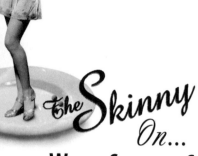

WHAT SKINNY GIRLS KEEP IN THEIR KITCHEN, IF ANYTHING

- Cookies your kids like and you hate
- Expensive condiments (make bland food taste like you ordered it at a fancy restaurant)
- Expensive mustard (kid yourself that it revs up your metabolism; also a great substitute for mayonnaise—well, not that great)
- Soup (tip: V8 when eaten with a spoon is almost gazpacho)
- Nonfat pineapple cottage cheese (add artificial sweetener and it's dessert)
- Very expensive fruit (but not too ripe—see The Skinny on Ripe Fruit vs. Nonripe Fruit)
- Diet Swiss Miss Cocoa (50 calories!)
- Extra-Crisp Wasa crackers (25 calories per ounce, more highly recommended than Ry-Krisp)
- Hard-boiled eggs (the whites are the meal, the yolk is the dessert)
- Edamane (just another name for boiled soybeans; at 130 calories per $\frac{1}{2}$ cup, they're a good substitute for nuts but not for lettuce sprouts)
- Tuna with mustard (fills up even "quantity" eaters)

190

- Herbal tea (makes you sweat uncomfortably, fills you up, and preparing it is an ordeal—you won't eat for at least another fifteen minutes)
- Baby carrots (we don't like them, but everybody else seems to so . . .)
- Celery (not a negative-calorie food, but you'd make diet history if you got fat on it)
- Fennel (sort of tastes good AND it's a diuretic!)
- Cantaloupe
- Grapefruit
- Nonfat yogurt (as a substitute for anything and everything, probably even Häagen-Dazs Chocolate Sorbet. And it's so good it doesn't need artificial sweetener.)
- Diet Popsicles (empty calories—our favorite kind)
- A handful of cashews (but no more)
- Cabbage soup (we don't believe the fat-burning theory, but it sure tastes good)
- Wine (keep drinking and you'll forget about food unless you're the type that remembers all too well)
- Fifty dark chocolate candy bars (see The Skinny on Oddball Tips)
- Clorox (to pour on all the above to make sure you don't eat it)

The *Skinny*

What to Do About Cellulite

Keep your pants on.

The *Skinny*

DIET BOOKS WE WISH WE'D WRITTEN

Hard as it may be for us to believe that there were other diet books written before, during, and probably after *The Skinny*, the evidence is incontrovertible. There are so many, in fact, that if you ate a page out of each of these, you'd feel bloated, even though paper has a very negligible caloric content. We vouch for none of them—they're just food for thought, which is the only kind of food that has absolutely no calories at all.

Eat Yourself Slim
Eat and Grow Thin
The Fat Boy's Book
The Joy of Slimming
Outwit Your Appetite
The Popcorn Diet
The Seventh-Day Diet
How I Lost 36,000 Pounds
Taming the Feast Beast
The Aztec Way to Healthy Eating
Calories Don't Count
News on Diet and Dietetics

Martin Luther and the Diet of Worms

Diet and Die

Diet Book for Junkies

Diet Book for Doctor, Patient, and Housewife: With Specimen Menus for One Week

Diet for Dogs

Diet for Epicures

Diet Without Despair

Dinnerology: Our Experiments in Diet from Crankery to Common-Sense

The Drinking Man's Diet

The Eating Man's Diet

Eating to Love: With Some Advice to the Gouty, the Rheumatic, and the Diabetic; A Book for Everybody

Enjoy Your Slimming

The Expense Account Diet

The Fat Boy Goes Poly-Unsaturated

The Fleshless Diet

Girth Control: For Womanly Beauty, Manly Strength, Health, and a Long Life for Everybody

The Hog and I: A Foolproof System for Controlling Weight

How Sex Can Keep You Slim

How to Reduce Your Weight or Increase It

It's In to Be Thin

It's More Fun to Be Thin

Man Alive: You're Half Dead

Martinis and Whipped Cream: The New Carbo-Cal Way to Lose Weight and Stay Slim

The No-Willpower Diet

The Non-Chew Cookbook

Pounds Off!

Reduce and Stay Reduced!

Slimming the French Way

Stay Slim for Life: A Diet Cookbook for Overweight Millions

The Teenage Surefire Diet Book

Victory Through Vegetables

Watching Your Weight—The Torah Way

What You Don't Know About Meat Eating

Shut Your Mouth and Save Your Life

Surplus Fat

The Skinny

ODDBALL TIPS

Here they are. A collection of favorite tips from our skinny friends. They work for them. And some of them may work for you:

- Sit-ups in the bathtub.
- Swallow a whole hard-boiled egg without any other food or liquid to wash it down. If all goes well, it will get stuck in your throat so that you can't eat anything else.
- Carry no cash on the street so you can't buy food.
- Brush your teeth early in the night so as not to eat afterward.
- Never eat a sandwich: It's stupid.
- Squirm during sex (imagine you are a snake and a stake has been driven through your body).
- Travel to a third world country—you will lose an easy 8 pounds.
- Smoke just two cigarettes a day.
- Take a smoking break during a meal.
- Keep a picture of a really fat guy like Tiny Hix on your refrigerator.
- Become a para-alcoholic and you will lose all interest in food.

- Buy dessert, take a bite, and throw the rest of it away.
- Give your food to your dog.
- Learn to be proud of throwing away food.
- Salt your dessert.
- Paint your fingernails so you can't use a fork or touch food—similarly, learn to do needlework.
- Drink three tablespoons of vinegar a day.
- Take a nap instead of bingeing.
- Nurse. ("I'd still be nursing my twenty-nine-year-old daughter if she hadn't rejected me at eight months," says our Skinny friend Lucille)
- Try new restaurants with a woman instead of a man because you will be able to order wisely.
- Steer your date to very expensive restaurants because the portions of food are smaller and there are more diet options on the menu.
- Encourage your husband to order food you don't like.
- Never eat breakfast—it's a waste of 500 calories.
- Eat dinner early with the children and old people and then never eat again until the next day.
- Beware of fruit juice. It has more calories than you think!
- Spend a lot of money on a personal trainer whom you can't cancel on so you won't be able to afford to skip your workout.
- Think of exercise as therapy, not fun.
- Exercise with kids so you can think it is "parenting."
- Eat Crystomint by the case (8 calories per mint).
- Eat chewy Ricola Mint Pearls. The minty taste makes it hard to eat anything else; plus you can't get it out of your teeth.

- Chocolate as an appetite suppressant.
- Chilled blueberries.
- Figs and water.
- Hot red pepper.
- Drink a concoction of lemon juice, cayenne pepper, maple syrup—it will make you so nauseous you can't eat.
- Keep only food that has to be cooked in your house.
- Shop for clothes instead of going to lunch.
- Have a single irreplaceable outfit that you have to wear to an important upcoming event.
- Arrive after nine P.M. when traveling—in most cities, you can't get food at that hour.
- One meal a day.
- Cut out the entrée, eat the rest.
- Order anything but eat only half of what's on your plate.
- If you want a cake, eat a cupcake.
- Indulgence days—"Donut Day," "Scone Festival"—followed by salad for ten days.
- Tylenol Sinus to give yourself a psychological jump start.
- Eat protein in the middle of the day.
- When you want to binge, pop a Valium and then turn on the TV and the urge to eat will pass.
- If you don't want to eat too much food, remind yourself that it will always be available.
- Go home to New Orleans and look at all the fat people.
- Buy cheap food—poor quality ice cream, bread, etc., contains less rich ingredients and more air.
- Drink all night so that you sleep all day (and therefore, don't eat).

- Salivation: chew your food slowly.
- Masturbation makes eating seem less urgent.
- Never eat anything that sticks to the plate when you run water over it. ("The Trickle of Water Test.")
- Try to get amoebic dysentery.
- Keep fifty dark chocolate bars in your refrigerator at all times so you never feel deprived.
- Visualize yourself thin every night as you go to sleep.
- Poach all food that can be poached.
- Eat all you want, but never swallow. Spit always.
- Hang upside down while you eat so the food won't stick. (We swear we know of someone who does this.)
- Go for medical tests: The anxiety of waiting for the biopsy report takes off 5 pounds.
- Have an illicit lover ("The Cheating Woman's Diet").
- Starve the evil you.

The Skinny

DIET TRUISMS

We can barely bring ourselves to do this, but we will now trot out the hoary old chestnuts of diet wisdom, for sentimental (and memory-jogging) reasons:

- Walk instead of drive, take the stairs instead of the elevator, park as far from the door as you can.
- Don't eat dessert. Not even a little.
- But if you're bound and determined to eat dessert, skip dinner.
- Never, ever, ever eat mayonnaise.
- Fish and chicken are better choices than beef and veal. Cut the large blobs of fat off of your steaks and chops and you will save some calories. Don't put butter on your filet mignon.
- Processed foods are almost always very high in calories.
- Don't eat potato chips or fried pork rinds.
- Don't eat anything fried, period.
- Fat-free is NOT calorie-free.
- Don't go grocery-shopping when you're hungry.
- Take small portions. Don't clean your plate.
- Learn to tolerate feeling a little hungry.

- If you think you're hungry, wait five or ten minutes and see if you stop feeling hungry. If you still are hungry, then eat.
- Don't keep fattening food in the house. Don't buy stuff for your kids that you like.
- Don't eat from other people's plates, ever.
- Sandwiches are stupid. Either eat the meat or eat the bread, not both.
- Salad dressing has a lot of calories.
- Soft drinks with sugar are incredibly high in calories. Learn to love NutraSweet.
- Water is a great filler. Stretch anything you can with it (soup, stews, etc.).
- Don't go to buffets. If you must go, don't eat anything.
- Order low-fat or low-calorie meals on planes.
- Don't eat in the car, in bed, on the street, in front of the refrigerator, out of containers, with your hands.
- Donuts are probably lost to you forever.
- Wear tight-waisted pants and skirts to dinners. When you start to suffocate, stop eating immediately.
- Don't believe your friends or your mother when they say you look too thin. They always will say you look too thin.

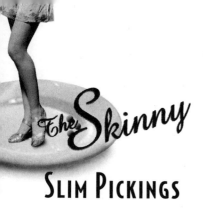

The Skinny

SLIM PICKINGS

Every diet book includes recipes. There is the obligatory sorbet, salad, and gazpacho. We have nothing against those recipes. They are standard diet food. But the following recipes are more . . . let's say, original.

FAKE CAKE

"WHILE THERE ARE MANY CHEESECAKES THAT TASTE BETTER, FEW ARE LESS CALORIC."

> 7 large eggs, separated
> ³/₄ cup cottage cheese
> ¹/₄ tsp cream of tartar
> 2 T sugar and 2 tsp Sweet'n Low
> Cinnamon to taste
> ¹/₂ tsp vanilla extract
> Lemon zest, as much as you want
> Pam or nonfat cooking spray

1. Separate the eggs. Put the whites in a large bowl. Put 2 yolks in another bowl.
2. Beat the egg yolks. Add the sugar, vanilla extract, cinnamon, and lemon zest.

3. In a blender (or Mixmaster), beat the cottage cheese until it is a creamy, lumpless soup-y liquid.
4. Combine the egg yolk mixture with the cottage cheese. Set aside.
5. Beat the 7 egg whites until they are stiff. Add the cream of tartar. Add the sugar and Sweet'n Low. (The sugar congeals the egg whites, but if you're desperate you can use only Sweet'n Low and sacrifice texture.)
6. Fold the yolk-cheese mixture into the egg whites. Add more Sweet'n Low if not sweet enough. Likewise, cinnamon.
7. Pour the batter into a Pam-sprayed 10-in. round spring-form pan
8. Bake at 350 degrees for forty minutes.
9. Cool at room temperature, then cool some more in the refrigerator.

Calories per cake: 464 (We're not going to make you feel bad by giving you the calorie count of a "serving size," thus implying that some people stop eating before they finish the entire cake.)

"I Can't Believe It's Not Grilled Cheese" and Technically it Isn't

Slather "I Can't Believe It's Not Butter" on the thinnest piece of bread you can find or a baked potato skin.

Stick in microwave oven for 30 to 40 seconds, or until the "butter" puffs up like open-faced grilled cheese.

Blot the grease off with a paper towel.

The "butter" will taste almost like Swiss cheese. In time, you will come to think it is delicious. If you are starving, you will think it is more delicious than cheese fondue.

Calories: Depends on your definition of "slather," but call it 80.

Emaciated Potatoes

Slice a potato into thin slices.
Place the slices on a paper towel.
Throw into the microwave for five to ten minutes or until the slices are chewy or crisp, depending on whether you are simulating french fries or potato chips.
Salt or season as desired.
This recipe also works well with zucchini, eggplant, or carrots.
Calories: Don't worry about it.

No-Crust Eggplant Pizza

Turn on your broiler.
Slice an eggplant lengthwise into $\frac{1}{2}$-in.-thick, wide pieces.
Definitely do not remove skin.
Spray the eggplant slices with Pam and arrange on a cookie sheet or pizza stone in a circle, overlapping the edges slightly.
Place under the broiler for five to eight minutes, or until the eggplant starts to brown and soften.
Remove cookie sheet from broiler.
Turn on oven to 500 degrees.

Layer the eggplant with pizza ingredients—no-fat tomato sauce, reduced-fat goat cheese, basil, onions, mushrooms, garlic.

Take off the sausage and pepperoni you just added and throw them away.

Get back to your pizza. Season liberally and return to hot oven. Bake 10 minutes.

Allow to cool slightly before cutting, and be prepared to use a knife and fork if there's a lot of topping.

Calories: Same as a low-fat pizza, minus the crust.

The Skinny

What, Finally, We Conclude

Contrary to what diet books tell you: There is diet magic. The magic is the phrase: Eat less food. The challenge is how to get yourself to eat less food, but no matter how much you manage to do it, eating less food, calorically speaking, will cause you to lose weight. The best way to do it is simply the way that works for you. The wide range of secrets and tips offered at the Skinny Lunches convinced us of this. You may be like many of the women we lunched with who are able to eat less by sticking to a low-fat diet, or you may be like other members of the contingent who thrive on a high-protein diet. You may be kin to the food writer who came to one of the lunches espousing the benefits of chewing gum and drinking lots of coffee. You may do well by padlocking your refrigerator after sundown. Or possibly, like the very slim travel writer who came to Lunch #9, you might be motivated by keeping gorgeous, skin-tight size 2 clothes in your closet. It may work for you to eat a huge breakfast or skip breakfast altogether (our lunch companions evenly split on this issue). Or perhaps you do best skipping food altogether until you get into bed late at night.

The specifics don't matter. The only important

thing is to figure out what works for you and your appetite and your particular psychological and physical wiring, and then stick to it until it stops working. Then you have to find another system, switch to it, and follow it until it stops working. There's no reason to think one particular diet is going to be the permanent answer to your thighs, and there's nothing wrong with working your way from one method to another. If low-fat worked for you for a while but doesn't work anymore, that's not failure—that's variety! Rigid adherence to prescribed diets that cease to work just doesn't make sense (except for ours, of course) because no specific diet works except one that you can live with. To get skinny, you need to understand yourself. What we've included in this book are some tricks and techniques that have worked for a lot of skinny women we know. One of them or probably even some of them will surely work for you.

Oh, by the way, calories do count. Really.

We have one final conclusion. We've been fat and we've been skinny and we've been several interim sizes and shapes, and—amazingly enough!—we conclude that we liked being skinny the most. Which is to say that at the end of the day, even if we're stuffed with celery sticks and Slim-Fast while yearning for chocolate and cream, we still feel that being skinny is worth the trouble if it means we don't need to use a shoehorn to get into our favorite pair of pants.

If you have your own skinny tips, please send them to skinnygirls@juno.com.

About the Authors

PATRICIA MARX has written for numerous TV shows, including *Saturday Night Live* and *Rugrats*. She is a regular contributor to the "Talk of the Town" (the *New Yorker*), *The New York Times Magazine, Vogue,* and many other magazines. She is also the author of several books, including *How to Regain Your Virginity, Now Everybody Really Hates Me, You Can Never Go Wrong by Lying,* and *Meet My Staff.* She was the first woman on the *Harvard Lampoon.* Patty has consumed more artifical sweetener than many laboratory rats.

SUSAN SISTROM leads many lives: writer, philosopher, food taster, and student of popular fashion. She lives and dines in New York

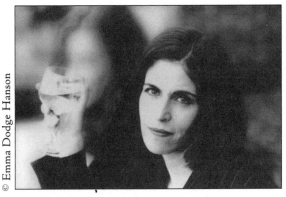

© Emma Dodge Hanson

Susan Sistrom, left, *and Patricia Marx*